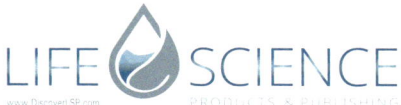

Copyright © 2018
Life Science Publishing & Susan Richardson, Brooke Sexton, & Bobbi Decker
1.800.336.6308
www.DiscoverLSP.com

Printed in the United States of America
10 9 8 7 6 5 4 3 2 1

© Copyright 2018. All rights reserved. No part of this book may be reproduced or transmitted in any form or by any means, electronic or mechanical, including photocopying, recording, or by any information storage and retrieval system, without permission in writing from the publisher.

Life Science Publishing is the publisher of this book and is not responsible for its content. The information contained herein is for educational purposes only and as a guideline for your personal use. It should not be used as a substitute for medical counseling with a health professional. The authors and publisher do not accept responsibility for such use.

Although the authors and publisher have made every effort to ensure the accuracy of the information contained in this book, we assume no responsibility for errors or omissions.

The essential and supplemental products discussed at length in this book are the sole product of Young Living Essential Oils, LC. The authors and publisher are completely separate entities from Young Living Essential Oils, LC. Products mentioned may be reformulated, discontinued, expanded, or enhanced by Young Living Essential Oils, LC at any given time.

Neither the authors nor the publishers advocate the use of any other essential oils without Young Living Essential Oils, LC's exclusive Seed to Seal® guarantee. Even minor changes in the quality of an essential oil may render it, at best, useless and, at worst, dangerous. The use of essential oils should be done with thorough study, watchful care, and judicious prudence.

Some of the content in this book is derived from the Essential Oils Desk Reference, one of the most widely sought, sold, and read essential oils books of all time. This content is used with written permission from the publisher. Life Science Publishing retains all rights to the content of both the Essential Oils Desk Reference and related volumes in this series.

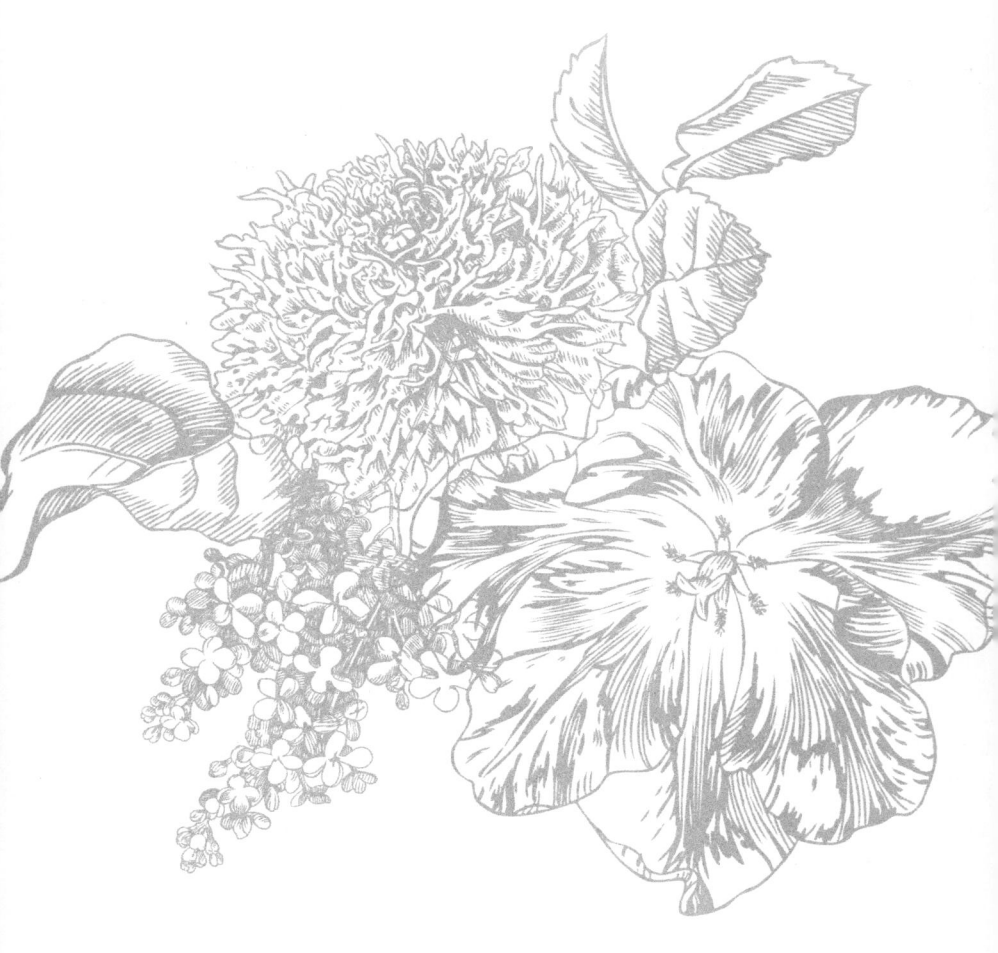

FOREWORD

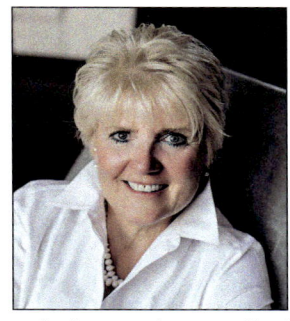

Now What? This book contains a four-month guide to supporting your wellness goals in a simple, easy layout aimed at one target—a completely new life for you.

The greatest tool we have for your health and wellness journey is ourselves. Knowledge is one thing, understanding is something else altogether. We can know many things, but if we do not understand what we know, all of our knowledge will be for naught. Wisdom is knowledge applied.

This little book explores some very practical ways in which our knowledge can simply be applied with the use of Young Living essential oils and supplements. It is very possible that the application of this little book could produce a better life for all of us—a life without dependency on exterior systems or aids, with no side-effects other than health and well-being.

What has been needed is some sort of simple system of immune support that the average person could access, understand, and apply.

Now What? is reliable information on a short, simple four–month plan of health maintenance that anyone can utilize. This book gives us a pacing guide on the road to individual good health and collective well-being. To create a better life, we must challenge ourselves to stay healthy and be in harmony with nature and with one's inner guidance.

Now What? educates you to the systems of the body and gives you choices to support and maintain all in a time period of just four months. This is a creative health program which may cleanse, build, and/or balance body systems to aid in greater daily health.

As Benjamin Franklin stated, *"An ounce of prevention is worth a pound of cure."* Self-education and self-awareness help us understand the relationship between man and nature, providing a therapeutic model—aromatherapy and whole based nutritional supplements which can strengthen and balance your body and sustain good health.

Marcella Vonn Harting, PhD

ABOUT THE AUTHORS

It's no secret that we love Young Living Essential Oils. But do you know what we love even more? Empowering people with a lifestyle that can authentically change the way they not only live life, but view it. Getting profound testimonies (daily) excites us! Wanting everyone to have a reliable tool to get them there drove us to write this book together...for you! Young Living is not just an essential oil company. We do not "do oils." This company, these EO infused products, and this journey are about achieving true health and wellness... physically, mentally, emotionally, and for us, even spiritually. If you are ready to explore a 4-month wellness plan, *Now What?* is your answer!

This is the first book of its kind... 100% FDA compliant, a Body Systems Approach to wellness which removes the guesswork and gives the avid business builder, or even the person who just wants to share with a few friends, a duplicatable system to share and personalize with others.

Susan Richardson

Bobbi Decker

Brooke Sexton

 Now What, Root Empowerment, LLC

 @NowWhat_YoungLiving

#RootEmpowerment #NowWhat #NowWhatYL

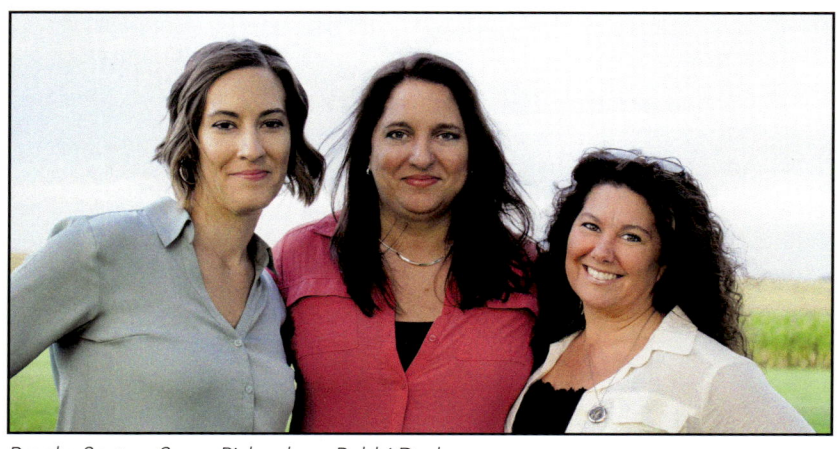

Brooke Sexton, Susan Richardson, Bobbi Decker

NOTE FROM A ROYAL CROWN

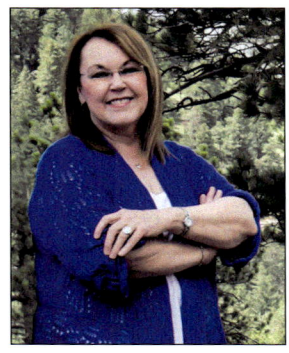

These three fabulous authors continue to change the lives of those around them in profound ways!

They came together to create this extraordinary resource making it simple to create a 4-month plan to optimize health and wellness!

This valuable book is a must-have for both new and seasoned Young Living members who want healthier and happier lives for themselves, their families, and their friends.

Vicki Opfer

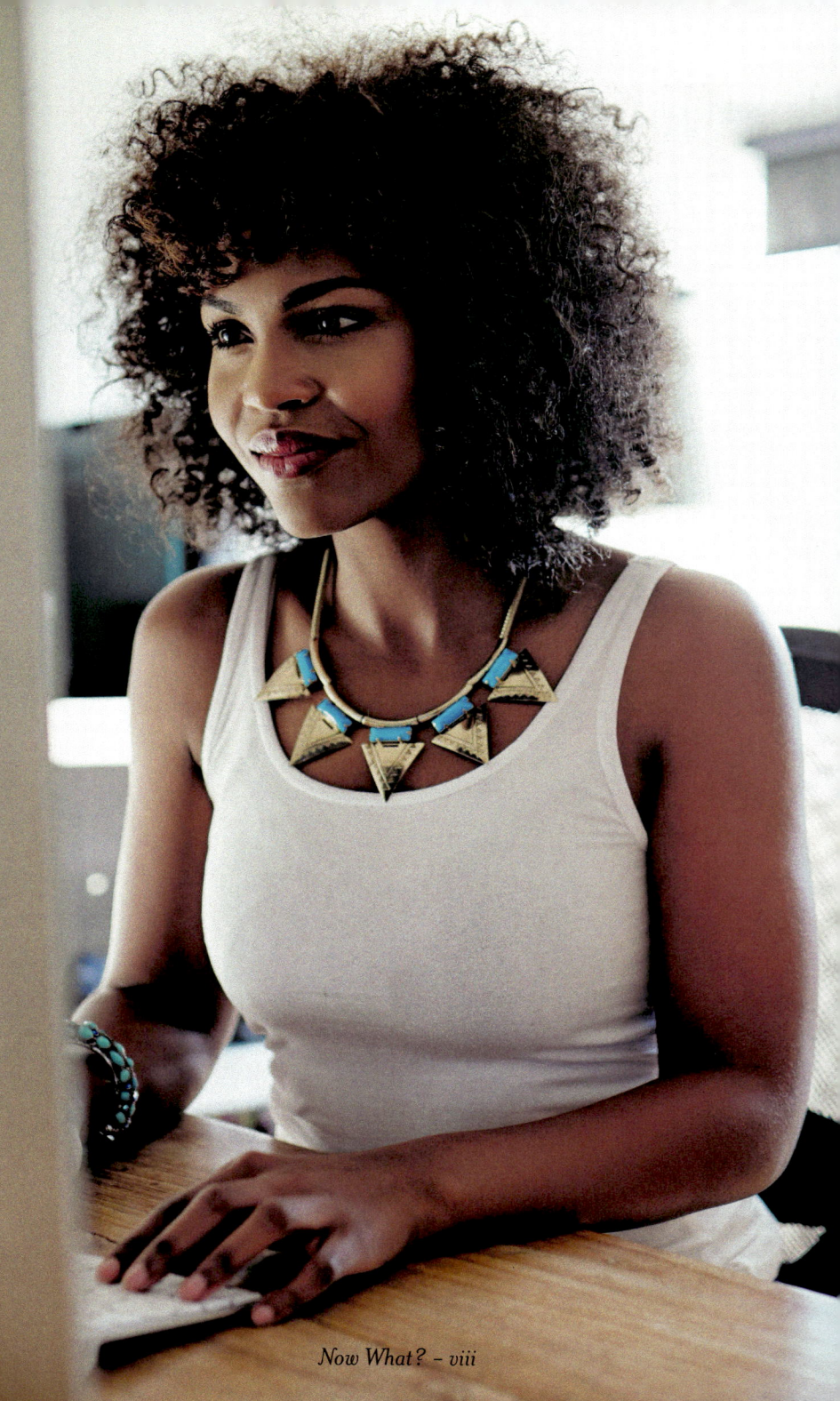

TABLE OF CONTENTS

Welcome 2
Essential Rewards 4
Cardiovascular/Circulatory... 6
Digestive/Excretory 8
Endocrine (Women) 10
Endocrine (Men) 12
Integumentary/Exocrine 14
Lymphatic/Immune 16
Musculoskeletal 18
Nervous System 20
Renal/Urinary 22
Reproductive 24
Respiratory 26
Feelings/Emotional Health 28
Anti-Aging 30
Antioxidant Support 34
Roller Ball Recipes 36
Diffuser Recipes 38
Sleep Support 40
Kids Support 41
Energy/Stamina 42
Brain Health 43
Baby Support 44
Summer Fun 45
Young Living Membership Benefits 46
Share More 48

WELCOME

We are so glad that you have decided to join us on your health and wellness journey. We are truly thrilled for each of you and your families!

This book is designed to empower you with scientifically validated information to assist you in designing a plan to meet your optimum health goals. Supporting each system of the body is a key component to reaching these goals. So, we have outlined these systems, along with nutritional information and suggestions, to help you plan out your first 4-months and beyond.

But before you do that, we recommend that you start a health journal. Simply write down how you feel today... emotionally, spiritually, psychologically, and physically. Stop and think about how your current health impacts all of the areas of your life. (Your family, job, energy, mood, relationships, mobility, stamina, etc.) Reflect in your journal upon how your life is impacted by this. Once you design and begin your wellness program, we want you to revisit your journal and track your progress. This is an important process as you begin to feel changes in your body, in your mood, and in your energy levels. Keep tracking your progress so you can evaluate your program and adjust
your wellness plan accordingly.

Your next step is to use the information in your journal to determine the first body system you want to target and support. Then go to that section of this book to review your product options and determine which products you are going to choose to establish your 4-month wellness plan.

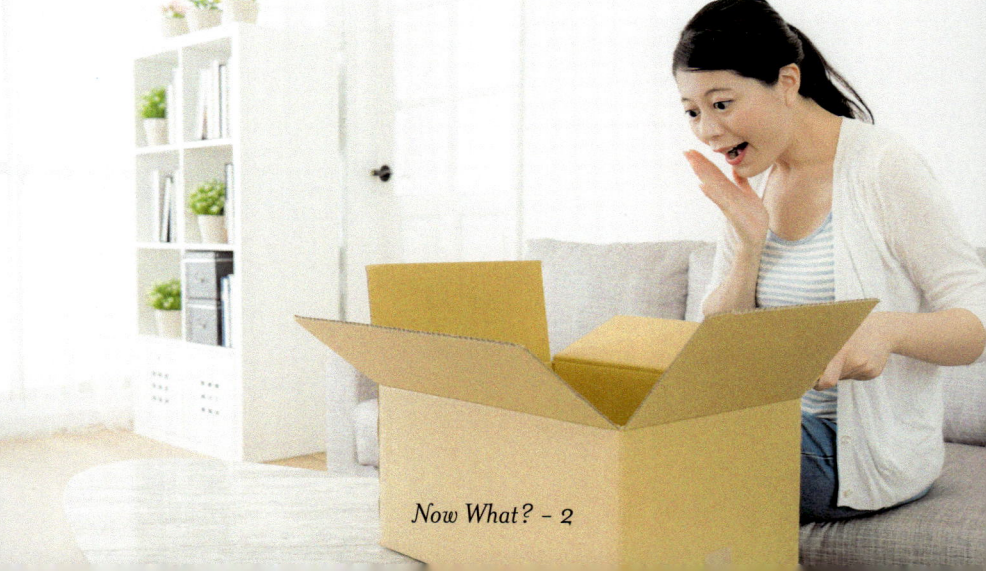

Now What? - 2

You will see throughout this book that many products are mentioned in various sections. This is because when using natural products, like Young Living's, they will help you target your health goals across multiple systems. When we fuel ourselves with proper nutrition and the power of essential oils, our bodies can self-regulate and heal themselves. Based on this, there is no need to discuss disease. Instead, create your 4-month wellness plan for your targeted body system, use the supplements and essential oils consistently, and then be amazed at how your body does its thing.

Remember that you may be addressing only one system of your body, but because you are increasing the nutrients you put into your body, you will be addressing every other system of your body simultaneously. So write down everything in your health journal, even if you think it is not related; you may be surprised at what you see.

Another important step on your wellness journey is to build a relationship with your sponsor. Your sponsor is someone who can help you design your 4-month plan and beyond. They can help you understand the most cost-effective way to implement your plan and earn free products at the same time; and there is even a business option if you so desire.

ESSENTIAL REWARDS

Young Living
Essential Rewards Program

An awesome auto-ship program full of great perks that does everything to support your wellness goals!

Exclusive Rewards Points
Earn points toward future purchases with every Essential Rewards order. The longer you are on Essential Rewards (ER), the more points you receive.

Months 1-3	Months 4-24	Months 25+
10%	20%	25%

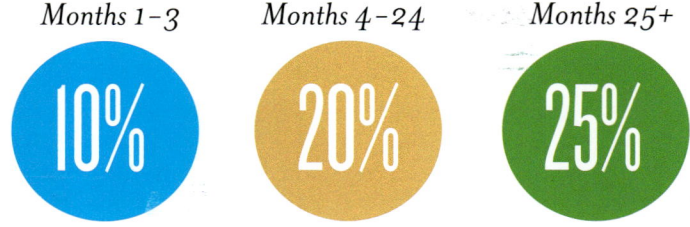

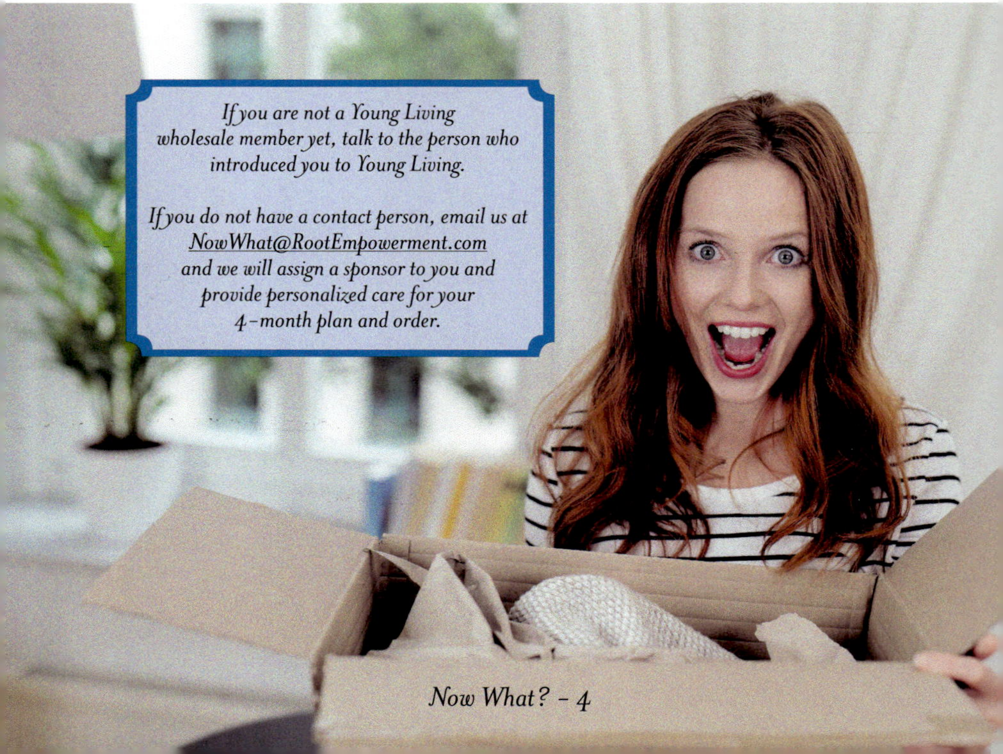

If you are not a Young Living wholesale member yet, talk to the person who introduced you to Young Living.

If you do not have a contact person, email us at NowWhat@RootEmpowerment.com and we will assign a sponsor to you and provide personalized care for your 4-month plan and order.

Discounted Shipping
Your ER order qualifies for discounted shipping rates which vary in price based on weight and shipping method.

Loyalty Gifts
Young Living rewards you for being a loyal member on the Essential Rewards program by sending you a free "Thank You" gift at your 3, 6, 9 and 12 month marks. After your first year, Young Living will send you a gift on your yearly ER anniversary.

Monthly Promotions
Each month Young Living offers product promotions. These promotions are free gifts that YL gives to us just for doing what we already do... order. The promotion is based on the PV (product value) of a single qualifying order and will be shipped automatically to you adding substantial value to your order. Check the virtual office for updated promotions.

Exclusive Bonuses
Essential Rewards members who place a minimum 100 PV order each month will also have access to exclusive income opportunities. Regardless, as to whether your goal is to cover your Young Living order OR to create a household income, talk to your YL sponsor about the compensation plan.

How to Sign Up for Essential Rewards

1. Become a Young Living Wholesale Member.
2. Personalize your order with your sponsor.
3. Complete the Essential Rewards Agreement.
4. Add products to your ER cart and choose a date you'd like it to process.
5. Start using your products consistently and watch your life change.

CARDIOVASCULAR/CIRCULATORY

This system circulates the blood around the body via the heart, veins, and arteries. This oxygenates the cells in your body, delivers nutrients, and carries away waste products. The heart is the body's hardest working organ.

Vitality Essential Oils
- Copaiba Vitality
- Frankincense Vitality
- Lavender Vitality
- Cinnamon Bark Vitality
- Marjoram Vitality
- JuvaCleanse Vitality
- Longevity Vitality
- Savory Vitality

Supplements
- Longevity
- Detoxzyme
- NingXia Red
- Master Formula
- MindWise
- MegaCal
- AgilEase
- Super B
- OmegaGize3

Complementary Products:
Stress Away, Frankincense, Lavender, Ocotea, Shutran, Aroma Life, Ylang Ylang, Cypress, Helichrysum, Essentialzyme, PowerGize, Kidscents Mightyvites and MightyZymes Chewable Tablets, SleepEssence, Pure Protein Complete

Cardio Raindrop:
Valor, Oregano, Thyme, Clove, Nutmeg, Goldenrod, Cypress, Aroma Life Essential Oils

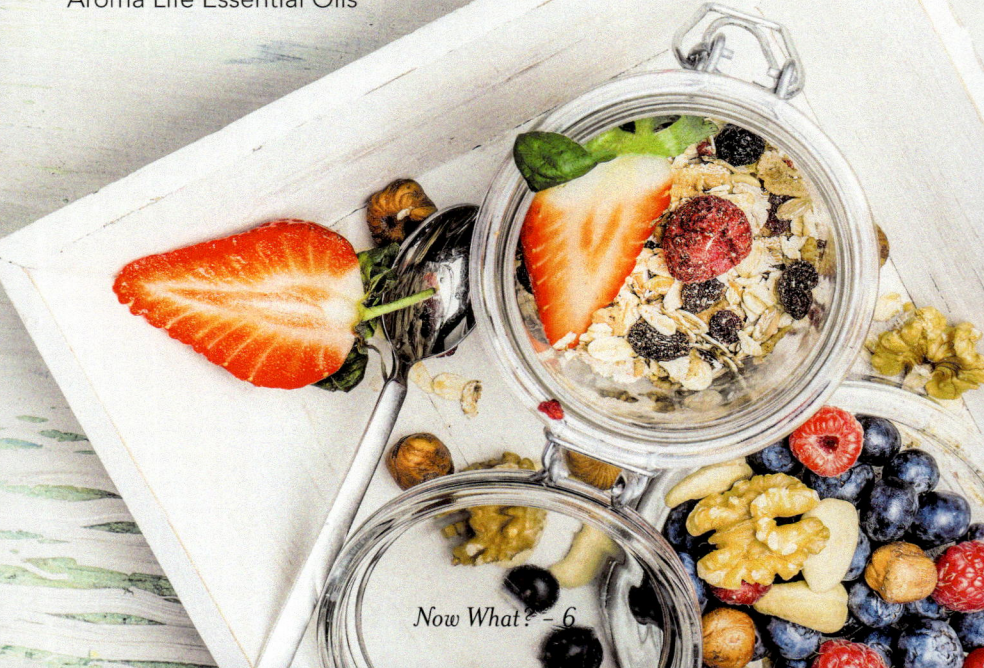

4-MONTH WELLNESS PLAN

Be sure to talk with your sponsor to personalize your 4-month plan and to calculate your product value (PV) to maximize your ER.

Month 1

Example: NingXia Red, MindWise, OmegaGize3, Cinnamon Bark Vitality, Ylang Ylang, Aroma Life

My Order: _____

_____

Month 2

Example: NingXia Red, MindWise, Longevity Softgels

My Order: _____

_____

Month 3

Example: NingXia Red, MindWise, Longevity Softgels, OmegaGize3

My Order: _____

_____

Month 4

Example: NingXia Red, MindWise, Longevity Softgels, Aroma Life

My Order: _____

_____

DIGESTIVE/EXCRETORY

This system consists of the mechanical and chemical processes that deliver the nutrients to our body and eliminate waste. These processes allow the body to produce energy and maintain normal cell function. Remember, all health begins in the digestive system.

Vitality Essential Oils
- Peppermint Vitality
- DiGize Vitality
- Nutmeg Vitality
- Lemon Vitality
- JuvaCleanse Vitality
- Tarragon Vitality
- JuvaFlex Vitality
- GLF Vitality
- Ginger Vitality
- Tangerine Vitality

Supplements
- NingXia Red
- JuvaTone
- Sulfurzyme
- Digest & Cleanse
- Cleansing Trio
- 5 Day Nutritive Cleanse
- ComforTone
- Essentialzyme
- Life 9
- Detoxzyme
- Balance Complete

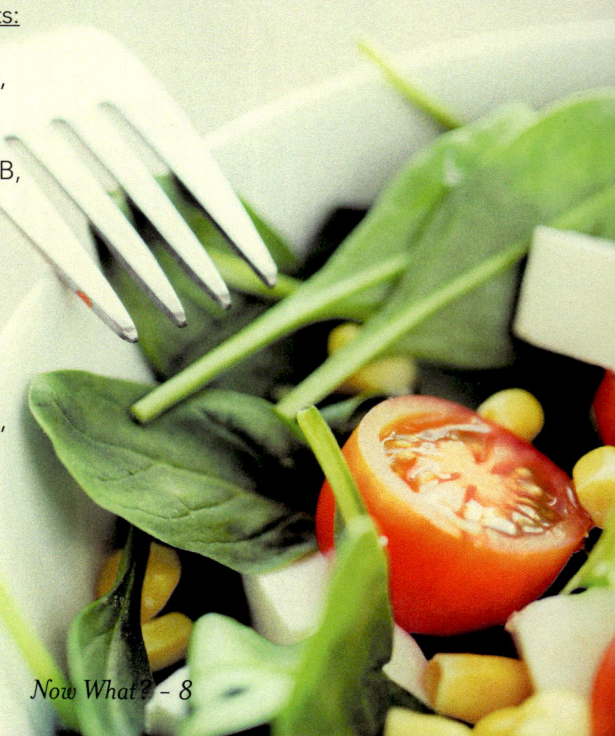

Complementary Products:
Peppermint, Sacred Frankincense, MindWise, AromaEase, SuperB, TummyGize, AlkaLime, DiGize, MultiGreens, K&B, OmegaGize3, JuvaPower, JuvaSpice, Essentialzymes-4

Digestive Raindrop:
Valor, Oregano, Thyme, ImmuPower, DiGize, Tarragon, Fennel, Cumin, Spearmint

4-MONTH WELLNESS PLAN

Be sure to talk with your sponsor to personalize your 4-month plan and to calculate your product value (PV) to maximize your ER.

Month 1

Example: NingXia Red, 5 Day Nutritive Cleanse, Sulfurzyme, Life 9, JuvaSpice

My Order: _____

_____

Month 2

Example: NingXia Red, Cleansing Trio, AlkaLime, Balance Complete, Life 9

My Order: _____

_____

Month 3

Example: NingXia Red, Allerzyme, Balance Complete, Life 9, Tangerine Vitality

My Order: _____

_____

Month 4

Example: Example: NingXia Red, Balance Complete, Alkalime, Life 9, Digize Vitality

My Order: _____

_____

Now What? - 9

ENDOCRINE (WOMEN)

This system provides chemical communications within the body. It encompasses the hormone-producing glands which cluster around blood vessels and release their hormones into the bloodstream. This system also includes the pituitary, adrenals, thyroid, parathyroid, ovaries, and pancreas.

Vitality Essential Oils
- Lemon Vitality
- Frankincense Vitality
- SclarEssence Vitality
- Sage Vitality

Supplements
- NingXia Red
- EndoGize
- PowerGize
- Thyromin
- CortiStop
- PD 80/20
- Super B
- Master Formula
- FemiGen

Complementary Products:
Frankincense, Peppermint, Myrtle, Sacred Frankincense, Progessence Plus Serum, Clary Sage, Dragon Time, Sensation, Lady Sclareol, SclarEssence, Transformation, Sacred Sandalwood, EndoFlex, Mirah Shave Oil

*Savvy Minerals Makeup—See pg. 33

Endocrine Raindrop:
Valor, Oregano, Thyme, Clary Sage, Progessence Plus, Endo Flex

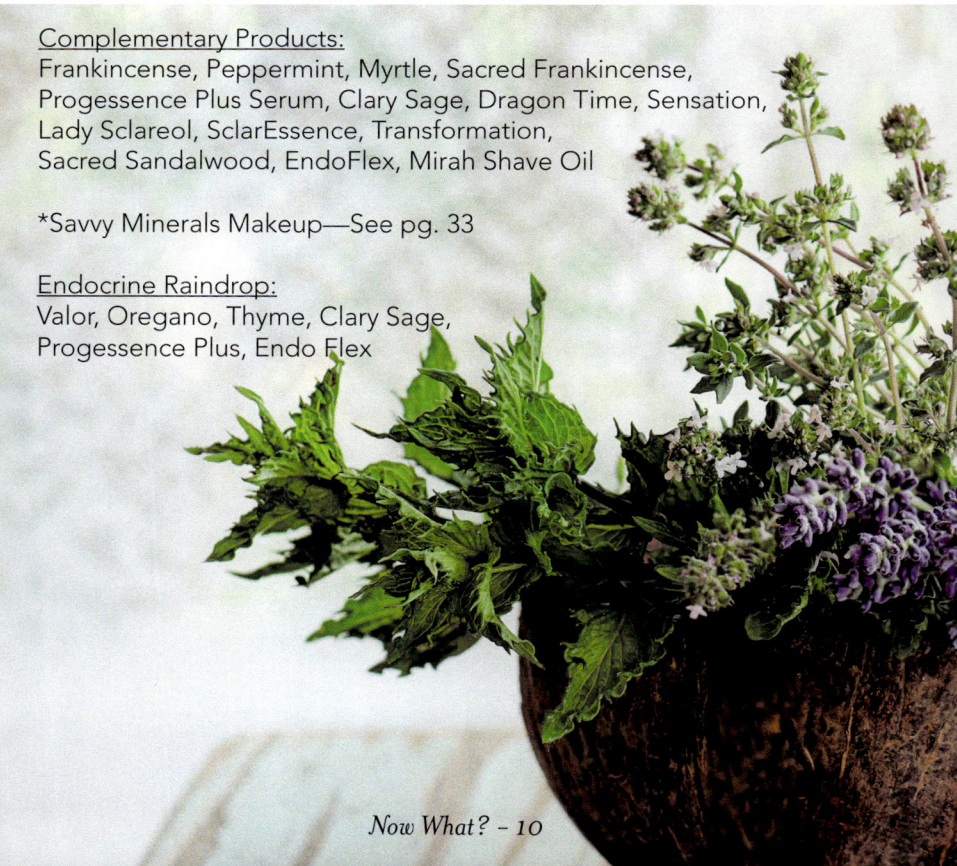

4-MONTH WELLNESS PLAN (WOMEN)

Be sure to talk with your sponsor to personalize your 4-month plan and to calculate your product value (PV) to maximize your ER.

Month 1

Example: NingXia Red, FemiGen, PD 80/20, Super B, CortiStop, Dragon Time Bath and Shower Gel

My Order: _____

_____

Month 2

Example: NingXia Red, Pure Protein Plus, FemiGen, PD 80/20, Super B, Clary Sage, EndoFlex, Mirah Shave Oil

My Order: _____

_____

Month 3

Example: NingXia Red, Pure Protein Plus, FemiGen, CortiStop, Super B

My Order: _____

_____

Month 4

Example: NingXia Red, Pure Protein Plus, FemiGen, PD 80/20, Super B, (Transformation 50+ or Progessence Plus)

My Order: _____

_____

ENDOCRINE (MEN)

This system provides chemical communications within the body using hormone-producing glands which cluster around blood vessels and release their hormones into the bloodstream. This is the hormone producing system of the brain. The thyroid is one of the most important glands for regulating the body systems.

Vitality Essential Oils
- Lemon Vitality
- Frankincense Vitality
- Longevity Vitality
- GLF Vitality
- Nutmeg Vitality

Supplements
- EndoGize
- PowerGize
- Thyromin
- Super B
- NingXia Red
- Master Formula
- Prostate Health

Complementary Products:
Frankincense, Peppermint, Myrtle, Sacred Frankincense, Sacred Sandalwood, Shutran, Shutran 3in1 Wash, Mister, Idaho Blue Spruce, EndoFlex

Endocrine Raindrop:
Valor, Oregano, Thyme, Shutran, EndoFlex

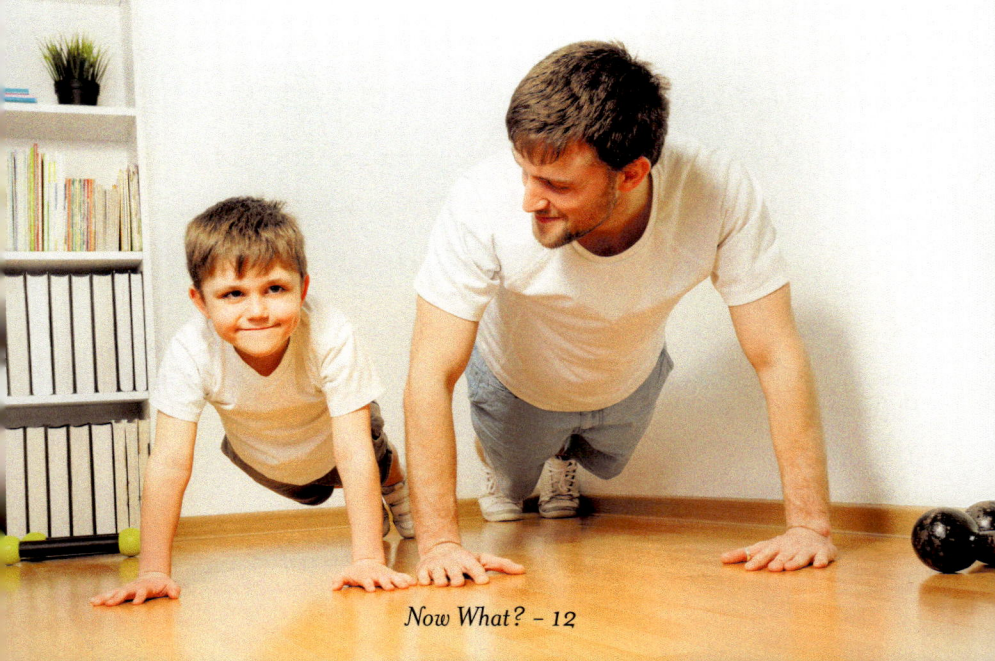

Now What? - 12

4-MONTH WELLNESS PLAN (MEN)

Be sure to talk with your sponsor to personalize your 4-month plan and to calculate your product value (PV) to maximize your ER.

Month 1

Example: NingXia Red, Master Formula, Prostate Health, Mister

My Order: _____

_____

Month 2

Example: NingXia Red, Master Formula, Prostate Health, Shutran

My Order: _____

_____

Month 3

Example: NingXia Red, Master Formula, Prostate Health

My Order: _____

_____

Month 4

Example: NingXia Red, Master Formula, Prostate Health; add Super B during the winter months.

My Order: _____

_____

INTEGUMENTARY/EXOCRINE

This system protects your body from environmental stressors and contains connective tissues, vessels, glands, follicles, hair roots, nails, sensory nerve endings, and muscular tissue. The skin is the largest organ in the body.

Vitality Essential Oils
- Lemon Vitality
- Frankincense Vitality
- Lavender Vitality
- Rosemary Vitality
- Carrot Seed Vitality
- JuvaCleanse Vitality
- Basil Vitality
- JuvaFlex Vitality

Supplements
- Sulfurzyme
- Master Formula
- AgilEase
- Super B
- NingXia Red
- Essentialzyme
- Detoxzyme
- ComforTone
- Life 9

Complementary Products:
Frankincense, Lavender, Sacred Sandalwood, Sacred Frankincense, Melrose, Gentle Baby, Tea Tree, Myrrh, Blue Cypress, Helichrysum, Rose, Veitiver, JuvaTone, JuvaPower, LavaDerm After Sun Spray, Mineral Sunscreen

See Young Living's Personal Care, ART Skin Care, and KidScents Product Lines.

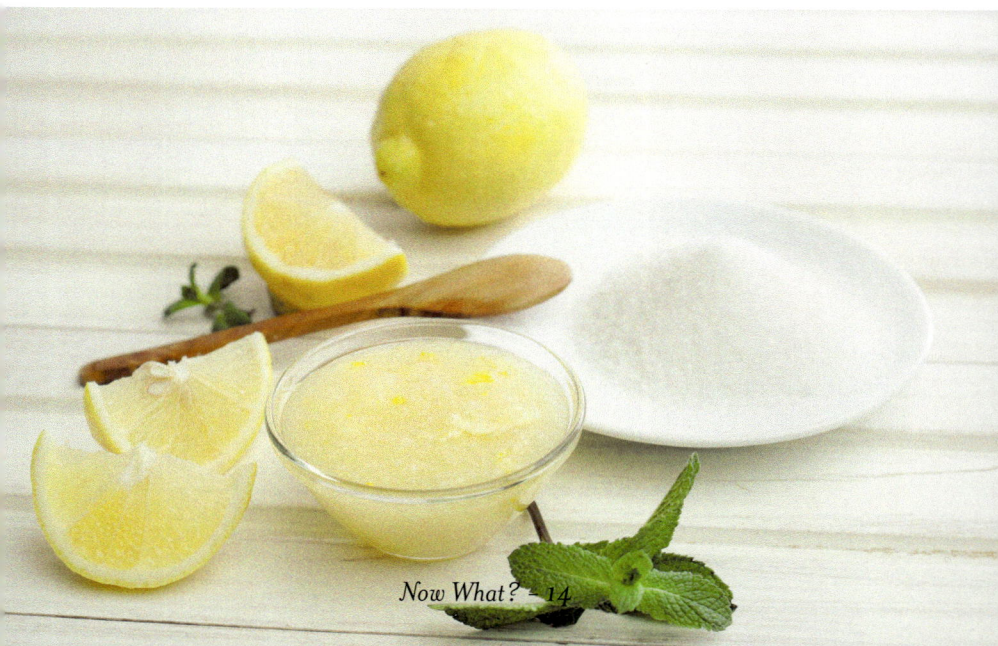

4-MONTH WELLNESS PLAN

Be sure to talk with your sponsor to personalize your 4-month plan and to calculate your product value (PV) to maximize your ER.

Month 1

Example: NingXia Red, Detoxzyme, Super B, Life 9, Shampoo/Conditioner, Orange Blossom Facial Wash, Cel-Lite Massage Oil

My Order: _____

_____

Month 2

Example: NingXia Red, Essentialzyme, Super B, Life 9, Lavender Bath & Body Gel, LavaDerm Mist

My Order: _____

_____

Month 3

Example: NingXia Red, Essentialzyme, Super B, Life 9

My Order: _____

_____

Month 4

Example: NingXia Red, Essentialzyme, Super B, Life 9, Copaiba Vanilla Shampoo/Conditioner, Orange Blossom Facial Wash

My Order: _____

_____

LYMPHATIC/IMMUNE

This system is a network of lymphatic vessels which defends the body against disease, fights infection, recycles plasma proteins, and drains fluid back into the circulatory system. This helps you stay hydrated and above the health line.

Vitality Essential Oils
- Thieves Vitality
- Frankincense Vitality
- Lavender Vitality
- Lemon Vitality
- DiGize Vitality
- Oregano Vitality

Supplements
- NingXia Red
- ImmuPro Chewable
- Inner Defense
- Life 9
- Super C Tablets
- Super C Chewables
- Longevity
- Digest & Cleanse
- MultiGreens
- Super B

Complementary Products:
ImmuPower, Aroma Life, Raven, En-R-Gee, Thieves Kit/Line, Exodus II, Cel-Lite Magic Massage Oil, Sacred Frankincense, Purification, Clove

Over the Counter:
Thieves Essential Oil Infused Cough Drops

Raindrop Technique:
Thyme, Basil, Peppermint, Oregano, Wintergreen, Cypress, Marjoram, Valor II, Aroma Siez, Ortho Ease Massage Oil, V-6 Vegetable Oil Complex

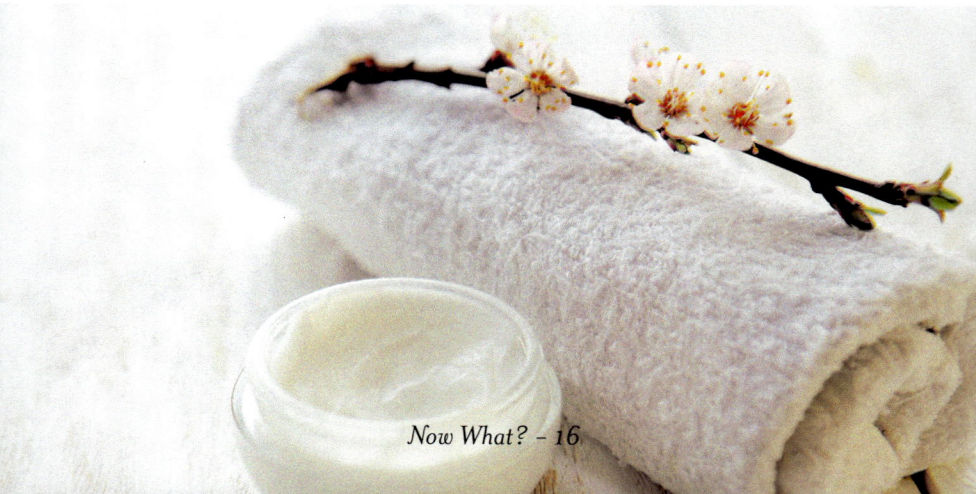

4-MONTH WELLNESS PLAN

Be sure to talk with your sponsor to personalize your 4-month plan and to calculate your product value (PV) to maximize your ER.

Month 1

Example: NingXia Red, Life 9, Inner Defense, Thieves Essential Rewards Kit

My Order: _____

_____

Month 2

Example: NingXia Red, Life 9, Inner Defense, Super C, MultiGreens

My Order: _____

_____

Month 3

Example: NingXia Red, Life 9, Inner Defense

My Order: _____

_____

Month 4

Example: NingXia Red, Thieves Essential Rewards Kit

My Order: _____

_____

MUSCULOSKELETAL

This system enables the body to move. It also supports your body and its organs, bones, joints, and ligaments.

Vitality Essential Oils
- Copaiba Vitality
- Frankincense Vitality
- Peppermint Vitality
- Lemongrass Vitality

Supplements
- NingXia Red
- AgilEase
- PowerGize
- OmegaGize3
- Super Cal
- Super Cal Plus
- Super B
- MultiGreens
- Master Formula
- AminoWise

Complementary Products:
Copaiba, PanAway, MindWise, Active & Fit Kit, Deep Relief, Wintergreen, Cool Azul Essential Oil Blend, Aroma Siez, Helichrysum, Dorado Azul, Ortho Sport Massage Oil, Pure Protein Complete, Marjoram, PD 80/20

Over the Counter:
Cool Azul Pain Cream

Raindrop Technique:
Thyme, Basil, Peppermint, Oregano, Wintergreen, Cypress, Marjoram, Valor II, Aroma Siez, Ortho Ease Massage Oil, V-6 Oil Complex (add Spruce, Helichysum, and Panaway to the rotation)

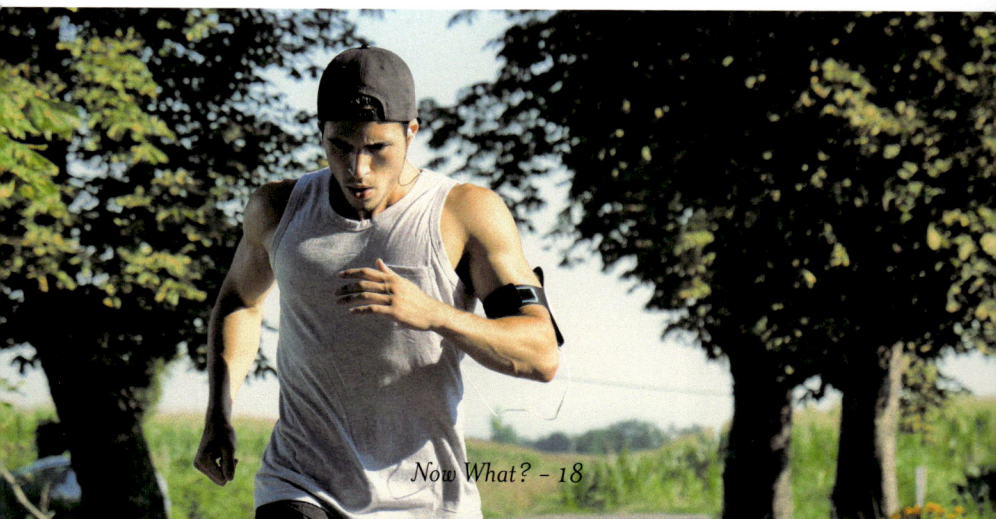

4-MONTH WELLNESS PLAN

Be sure to talk with your sponsor to personalize your 4-month plan and to calculate your product value (PV) to maximize your ER.

Month 1

Example: NingXia Red, AgilEase, PowerGize, OmegaGize 3

My Order: _____

Month 2

Example: NingXia Red, MindWise, OTC Cool Azul Pain Cream, Copaiba Vitality

My Order: _____

Month 3

Example: NingXia Red, AgilEase, PowerGize, OmegaGize 3

My Order: _____

Month 4

Example: NingXia Red, MindWise, OTC Cool Azul Pain Cream, Copaiba Vitality

My Order: _____

NERVOUS SYSTEM

This system collects and processes information from the nerves in the brain. The autonomic nervous system controls involuntary activities such as heartbeat, breathing, digestion, glandular activities and the blood vessels. This system is greatly affected by the digestive system.

Vitality Essential Oils
- Frankincense Vitality
- Lavender Vitality
- Rosemary Vitality
- Lemon Vitality

Supplements
- NingXia Red
- NingXia Nitro
- MindWise
- OmegaGize 3
- MegaCal
- Mineral Essence
- Super C Tablets/Chewables
- MultiGreens
- Master Formula

Complementary Products:
Reconnect Kit, Melissa, Helichrysum, Clarity, Brain Power, KidScents MightyVites/Zymes, Super B, Personal Care Products, Rosemary, Cedarwood, Sleep Essence

Raindrop/NAT Technique:
Cardamom, Peppermint, Clarity Blend, M-Grain, Stress Away, Frankincense, Sacred Sandalwood, Vetiver, Valerian, Valor, Cedarwood, RutaVaLa

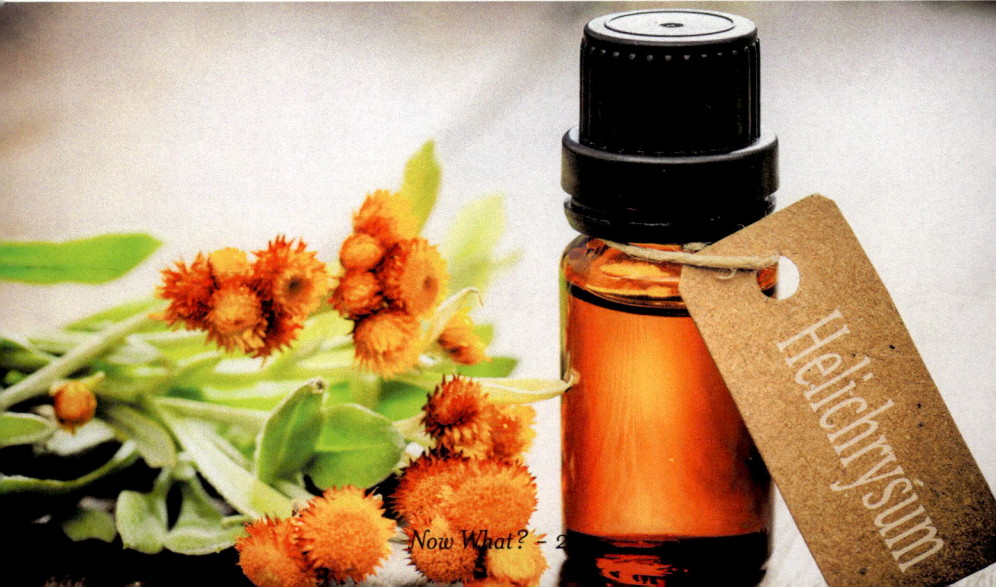

4-MONTH WELLNESS PLAN

Be sure to talk with your sponsor to personalize your 4-month plan and to calculate your product value (PV) to maximize your ER.

Month 1

Example: MindWise, NingXia Red, NingXia Nitro, OmegaGize 3, BrainPower, Mineral Essence

My Order: _____

_____

Month 2

Example: NingXia Red, Thieves Cleaning Kit, Shampoo, Conditioner, Handsoap, Rosemary Vitality

My Order: _____

_____

Month 3

Example: MindWise, NingXia Red, Sacred Frankincense, NingXia Nitro

My Order: _____

_____

Month 4

Example: MindWise, NingXia Red, NingXia Nitro, OmegaGize 3, BrainPower, Mineral Essence

My Order: _____

_____

Now What? –

RENAL/URINARY

This system is where the kidneys filter the blood and remove waste products and maintain normalized blood pressure. When you stay above the health line, your kidneys filter over 200 quarts of blood every day and remove more than 2 quarts of waste that flow through the bladder.

Vitality Essential Oils
- Lemon Vitality
- Frankincense Vitality
- DiGize Vitality
- GLF Vitality
- Grapefruit Vitality
- Oregano Vitality

Supplements
- NingXia Red
- K & B
- Digest & Cleanse
- Inner Defense
- AlkaLime
- Balance Complete
- Mineral Essence
- ImmuPro
- AgilEase
- Essentialzyme

Complementary Products:
Juniper, Eucalyptus Blue, JuvaCleanse, JuvaTone, Clove, Rosemary, Thieves, Copaiba, Life 9

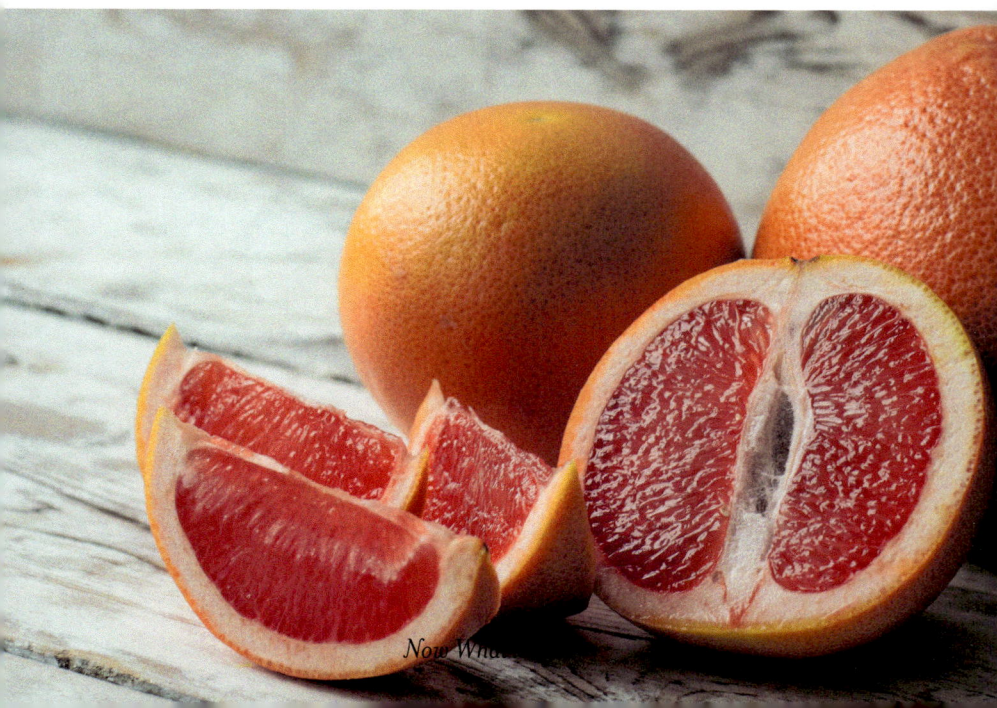

4-MONTH WELLNESS PLAN

Be sure to talk with your sponsor to personalize your 4-month plan and to calculate your product value (PV) to maximize your ER.

Month 1

Example: NingXia Red, K&B, Balance Complete, ImmuPro, Inner Defense, Life 9

My Order: _____

_____

Month 2

Example: NingXia Red, K&B, Balance Complete, ImmuPro, Inner Defense, Life 9, Lemon Vitality, Grapefruit Vitality

My Order: _____

_____

Month 3

Example: NingXia Red, K&B, Balance Complete, ImmuPro, Inner Defense, Life 9, Lemon Vitality, Grapefruit Vitality

My Order: _____

_____

Month 4

Example: NingXia Red, K&B, Balance Complete, ImmuPro, Inner Defense, Life 9, Lemon Vitality, Grapefruit Vitality

My Order: _____

_____

REPRODUCTIVE SYSTEM

This system includes your sex organs which are required for the production of offspring.

Vitality Essential Oils
- Frankincense Vitality
- Lavender Vitality
- EndoFlex Vitality
- Sage Vitality
- Nutmeg Vitality

Supplements
- NingXia Red
- MultiGreens
- FemiGen
- PowerGize
- Prostate Health
- PD 80/20
- EndoGize
- Master Formula
- Sulfurzyme
- Thyromin

Complementary Products:
Ultra Young + Oral Spray with DHEA, Shutran, Progessence Plus Serum, Protec, Clary Sage, SclarEssence, Mister, Lady Sclareol, Live with Passion, Ylang Ylang, Sensation, Sensation Message Oil, Oola Family, Oola Fun, Jasmine, Stress Away, Sacred Frankincense, Goldenrod, Idaho Blue Spruce, Rose

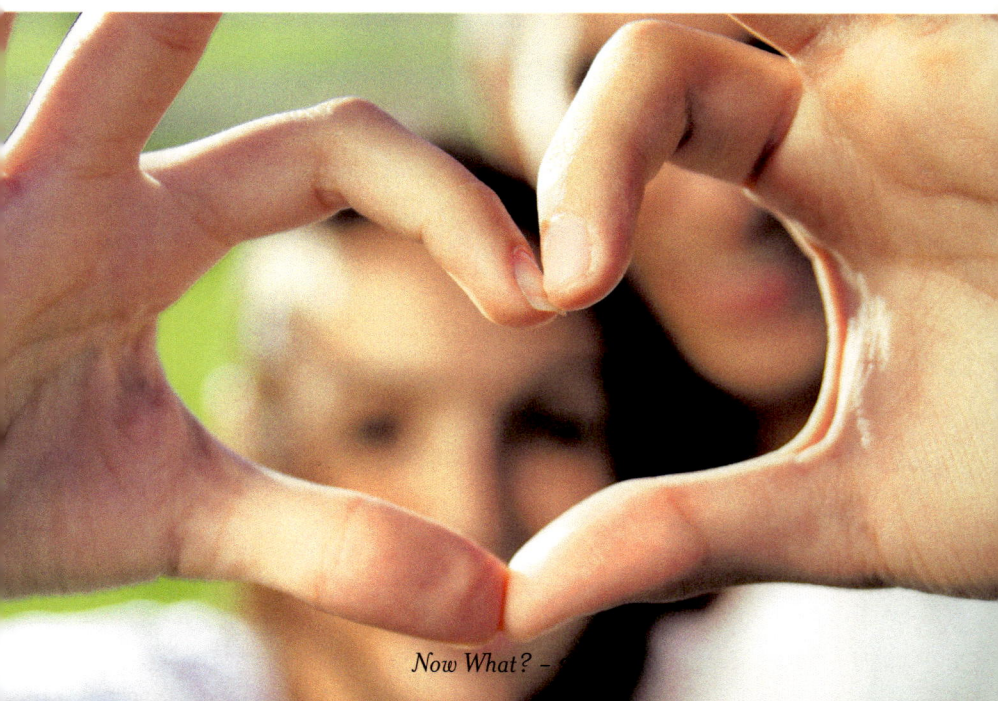

Now What?

4-MONTH WELLNESS PLAN

Be sure to talk with your sponsor to personalize your 4-month plan and to calculate your product value (PV) to maximize your ER.

Month 1

Example: NingXia Red, Master Formula, Shutran or Mister for men, FemiGen for women

My Order: _____

_____

Month 2

Example: NingXia Red, Master Formula, Prostate Health for men, PD 80/20 for women

My Order: _____

_____

Month 3

Example: NingXia Red, Master Formula, Prostate Health for men, PD 80/20 for women

My Order: _____

_____

Month 4

Example: NingXia Red, Master Formula, Prostate Health for men, PD 80/20 for women

My Order: _____

_____

RESPIRATORY SYSTEM

This system carries oxygen-rich air to your lungs and carbon dioxide and waste gas out of your lungs. This includes your nose and linked air passages, mouth, larynx, trachea, and bronchial tubes.

Vitality Essential Oils
- Frankincense Vitality
- Peppermint Vitality
- Thieves Vitality
- Lemon Vitality

Supplements
- NingXia Red
- ICP
- MultiGreens
- ImmuPro
- Inner Defense
- Life 9
- Detoxzyme
- Essentialzyme
- Super C Tablets/Chewables
- Sulfurzyme

Complementary Products:
Myrrh, RC, Raven, Ravintsara, Breathe Again, Eucalyptus Blue, Eucalyptus Radiata, Sacred Mountain, Palo Santo, Dorado Azul, Idaho Ponderosa Pine, Thieves Kit/Line/Oral Care, Purification, Myrtle, Rosemary, German Chamomile, Melissa, Personal Care Products, JuvaPower, AromaLux/AromaDome combo

Over the Counter:
Thieves Essential Oil Infused Cough Drops

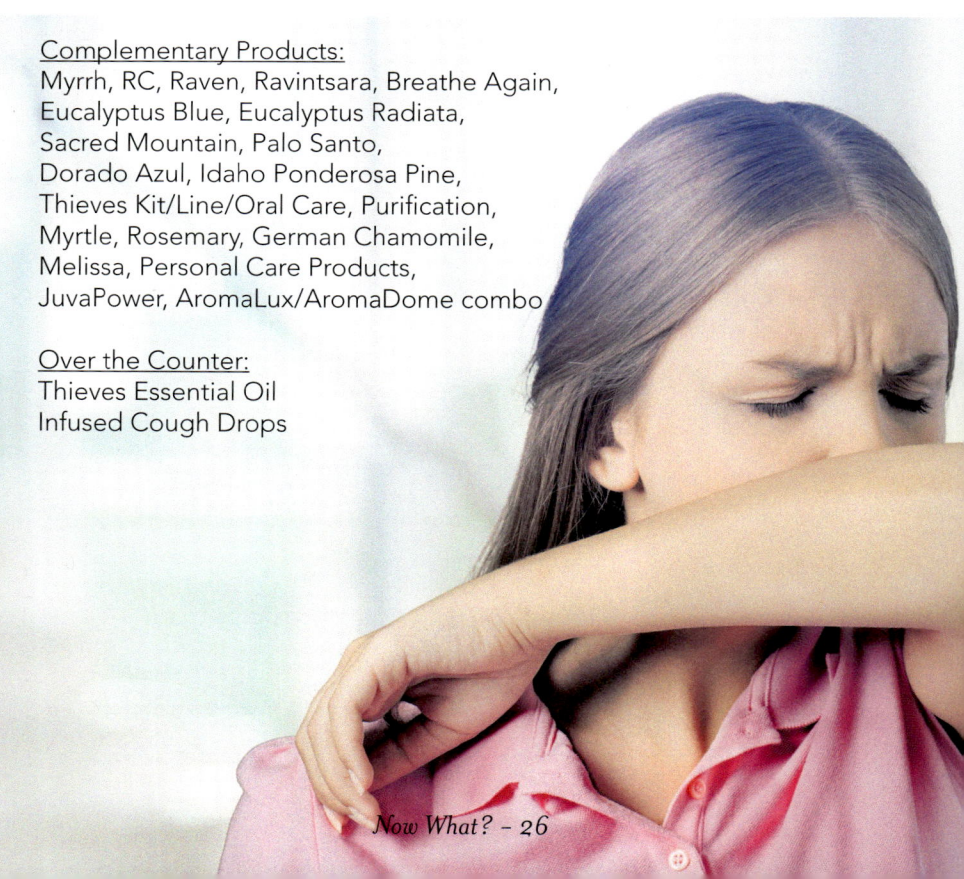

4-MONTH WELLNESS PLAN

Be sure to talk with your sponsor to personalize your 4-month plan and to calculate your product value (PV) to maximize your ER.

Month 1

Example: NingXia Red, MultiGreens, Inner Defense, Life 9, and Thieves Cleaning Kit

My Order: _____

_____

Month 2

Example: NingXia Red, MultiGreens, Inner Defense, Life 9, and RC

My Order: _____

_____

Month 3

Example: NingXia Red, MultiGreens, Inner Defense, Life 9, Thieves Vitality, Lemon

My Order: _____

_____

Month 4

Example: NingXia Red, MultiGreens, Inner Defense, Life 9, Eucalyptus

My Order: _____

_____

FEELINGS/EMOTIONAL HEALTH

Young Living Essential Oils and Blends can stimulate emotional health.

Awaken
A blend of 5 essential oil blends formulated to "awaken" your inner awareness. Understanding yourself is a great beginning to transforming your life.

Grounding
An empowering earthy scent that helps to provide stability and balance during any environmental or internal chaos. Grounding helps you relax and cope with reality with a positive attitude.

Forgiveness
Is very soothing and uplifting. This blend may enhance your ability to release memories that no longer serve you so that you can move on to a happier, more productive life.

Harmony
Promotes physical and emotional harmony. This relaxing essential oil blend helps us to balance and renew our sense of self while contributing to feelings of well-being.

Inner Child
Nurtures your inner child and helps you find inner strength. Individuals who have experienced traumatic experiences in their childhood have found that this sweet aroma helps to balance their emotions.

Joy
Promotes charismatic energy and brings joy to the heart when experiencing the everyday blues. Wear this blend as perfume with purpose that inspires romance, happiness and uplifted emotions.

Release
Stimulates feelings of peace, harmony, and balance in the mind and body while facilitating the ability to release anger and frustration. Repressed negative emotions lie at the root of many health concerns.

Sara
A powerful blend that was formulated to help soothe deep emotional wounds and release emotional baggage.

Trauma Life
Is made to guide you on your healing journey, to aide in the release of buried emotions that can pop up at the most inopportune times. This blend is both calming and grounding and a must-have for anyone working on issues from the past.

White Angelica
For those times when you know you will be exposed to stress-filled environments and negative people. Diffuse it or wear it like a protective shield. This oil cultivates and strengthens feelings of security.

Feelings Kit
A powerhouse of six essential oil blends to address everything listed above and more. Includes Valor, Harmony, Forgiveness, Inner Child, Release, and Present Time.

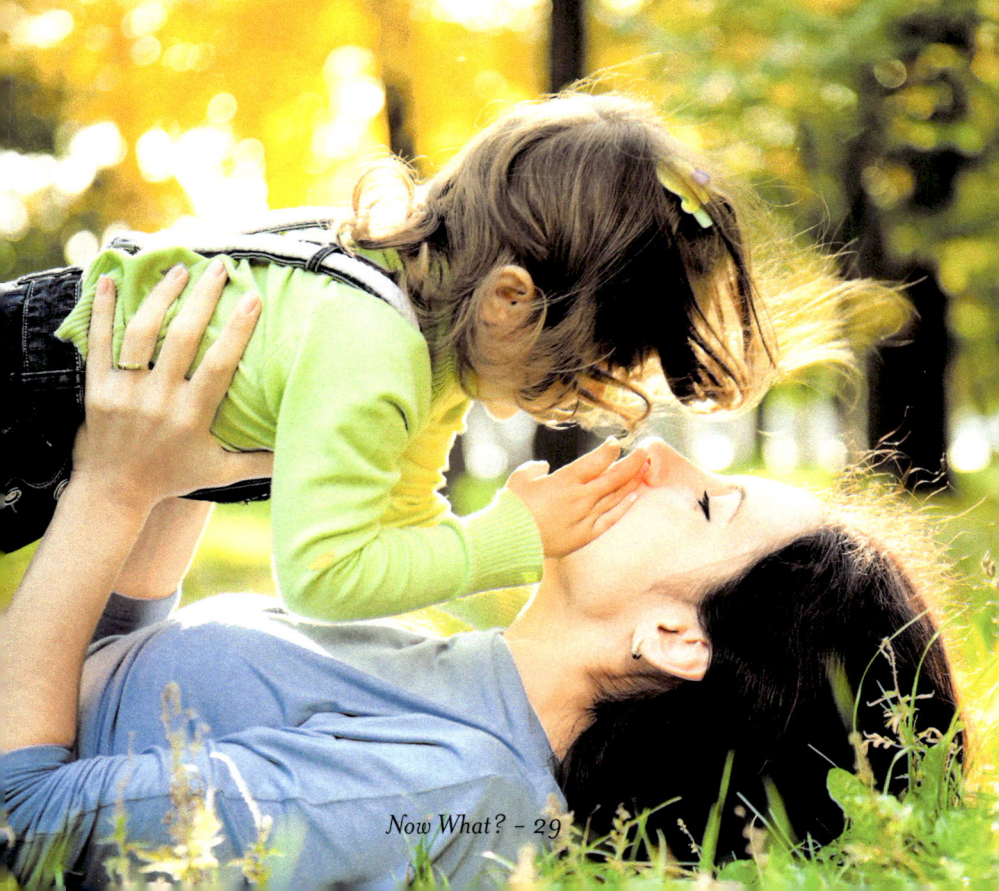

ANTI-AGING

You can erase the signs of aging by using the Young Living anti-aging line. The ART system is infused with essential oils to imbue your skin with vibrancy and vitality.

Rose Ointment
Gives new life to dry skin by improving the feel and appearance. Features Tea Tree and Rosewood essential oils to soothe rough, irritated skin.

Sheerlumé
Contains a proprietary blend of alpine botanicals and pure essential oils that will brighten sallow tones, and balance your complexion so you don't need chemical laden products to make you feel more confident and beautiful.

L'Brianté
These lip gloss/essential oil scent duos are a perfect addition to your makeup travel bag. Two products in one to make more room for your other must haves.

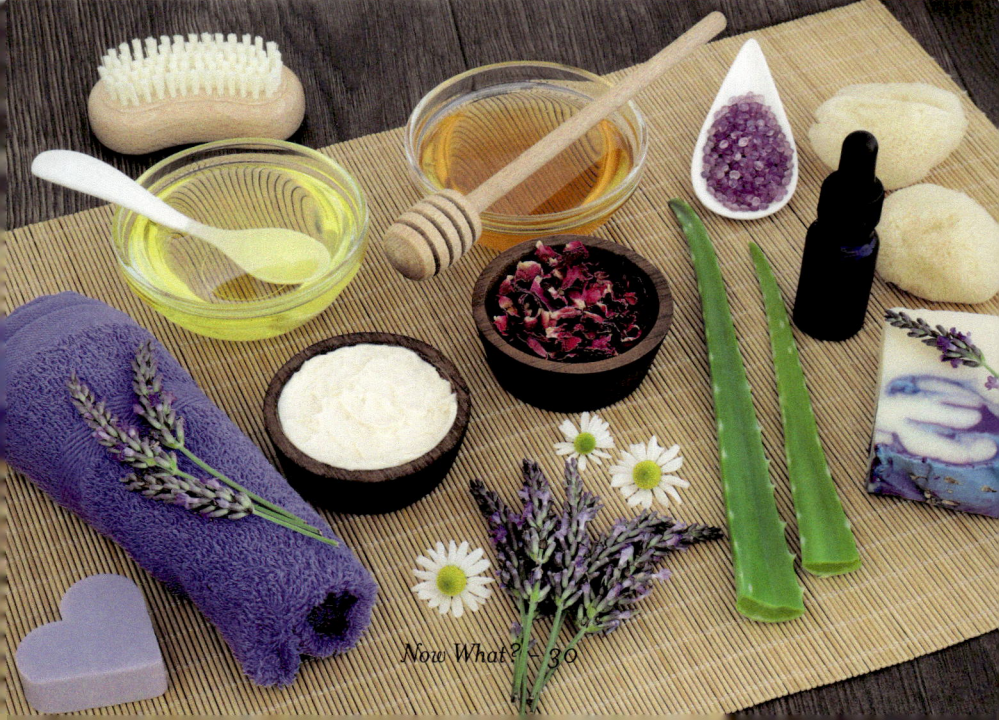

Satin Facial Scrub Mint
A water-based exfoliant containing a unique combination of jojoba oil, mango butter, MSM, aloe, and Peppermint essential oil. Keep this natural scrub in the shower to use regularly to minimize the appearance of pores and brighten your skin.

Orange Blossom Facial Wash
Contains MSM and Lavender essential oil to soften and support sensitive skin. This is a very gentle soap-free cleanser which helps remove impurities without stripping away your natural balance of oils.

Young Living's ART Skin Care System
Infused with essential oils to safely and effectively cleanse, tone, and moisturizes your face. When properly hydrated, our skin cells naturally regenerate which not only brightens our complexion, but keeps us looking younger.

ART Renewal Serum
Contains orchid extract. Essential oils are gentle on sensitive areas of your face. This serum is formulated to nourish, hydrate, and help maintain a youthful appearance.

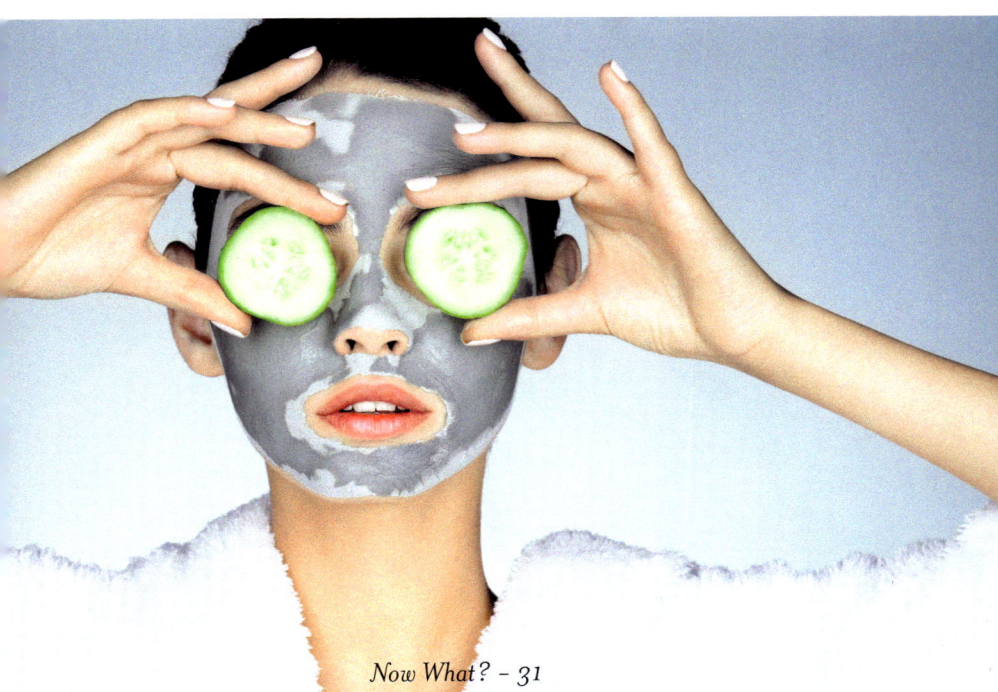

ANTI-AGING (CONTINUED)

Boswellia Wrinkle Cream
Contains Frankincense and Sandalwood straight from our farms. This moisturizer nourishes and soothes the skin while minimizing shine. It also contains MSM that supports healthy collagen to improve skin firmness and the appearance of wrinkles and fine lines.

Sandalwood Moisture Cream
A premium hydrating moisturizer infused with Young Living's pure Sandalwood essential oil. It also contains Rosemary, Myrrh, Geranium, Wolfberry Seed oil and other botanicals to support and hydrate more mature skin.

Shutran Aftershave Lotion
100% plant-based and quick absorbing. It soothes, cools, and calms skin after shaving. Made with Shutran essential oil blend, organic coconut oil, argan oil, jojoba oil, witch hazel extract, dandelion root extract, and aloe vera. This is the perfect moisturizing companion to Young Living's Shutran Shave Cream and essential oil blend for men.

ART® Creme Masque
Deeply moisturizing for your skin. Infused with pure essential oils and other luxurious botanicals this masque is formulated to
restore the look of youthfulness to the skin.
Gentle enough for all skin types.

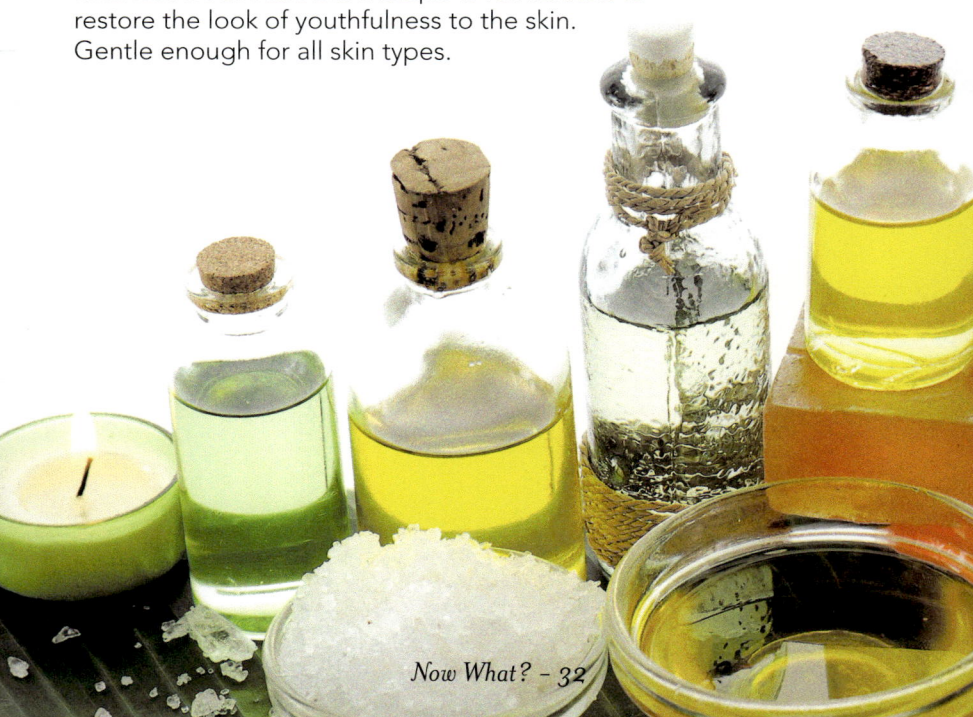

Savvy Minerals Makeup
Formulated with the same unwavering standards embracing the seed to seal promise. Free of synthetics and cheap fillers, the natural and non-toxic makeup line stands alone in quality and purity while supporting our health and maintaining body system integrity.

ART Beauty Serum
Formulated for dry skin. Infused with essential oils like Blue Cypress, Lavender, Cedarwood, Myrrh, Clove, Sandalwood and Wolfberry Seed oil which work synergistically to support and restore the skin's natural moisture balance.

LavaDerm
Cooling mist that contains Lavender, Helichrysum, aloe and ionic trace minerals to soothe and rejuvenate skin when overexposed to the elements.

Wolfberry Eye Cream
A water-based moisturizer. Containing the anti-aging and skin-conditioning properties Coriander, Roman Chamomile, Frankincense, mango seed butter and Wolfberry Seed oil; this cream soothes tired eyes and minimizes the appearance of fine lines.

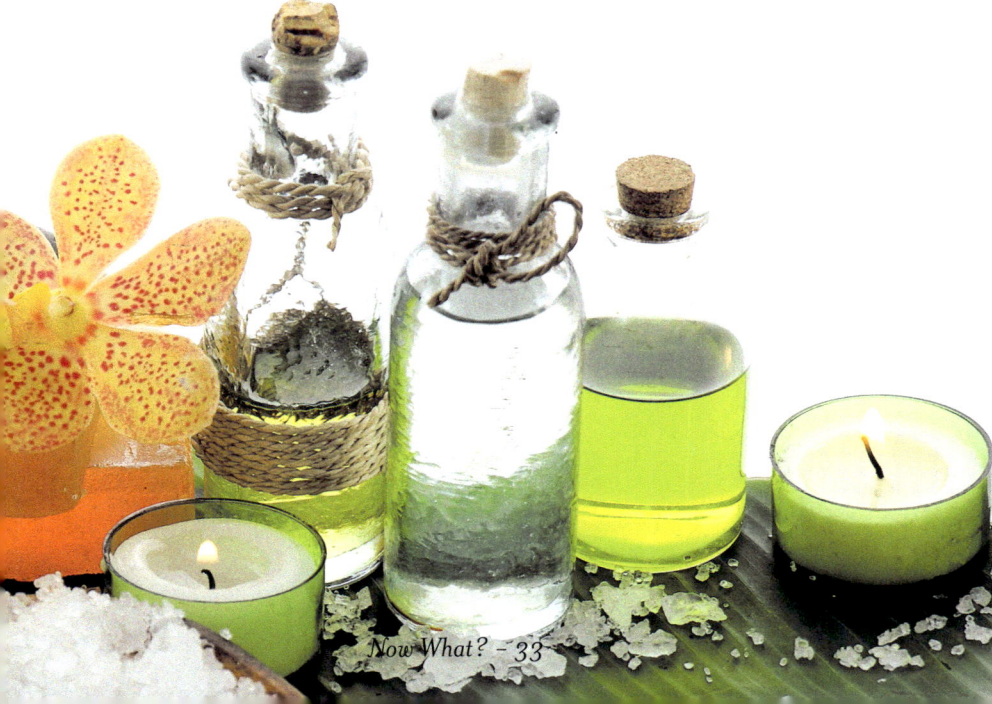

ANTIOXIDANT SUPPORT

Longevity Softgels
Contains a proprietary blend of fat-soluble antioxidants which helps to strengthen the body's systems response to the damaging effects of free radicals, aging, diet, and other everyday environmental stressors. It contains Clove oil which is known to be nature's strongest antioxidant.

Longevity Essential Oil Blend
Contains oils that rank among the most powerful antioxidants known. Antioxidants help to neutralize free radicals and lessen oxidative damage. Longevity contains ingredients that score a very high 1,500,000 on the ORAC scale.

Mineral Essence
Mineral Essence supports a healthy immune system and contains an ionic mineral complex infused with invigorating essential oils.

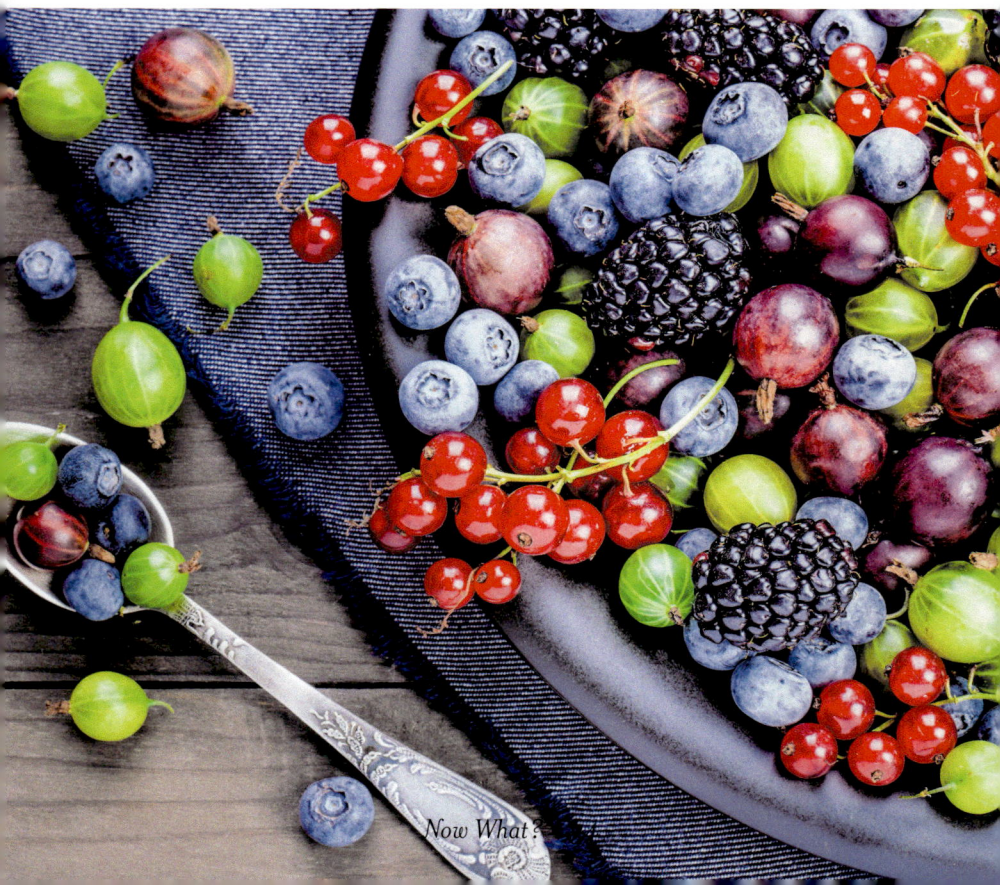

NingXia Red
NingXia Red combines Wolfberry fruit puree, blueberry, plum, cherry, aronia and pomegranate juices with 100% pure essential oils in a powerful, whole-body nutrient dense infusion. The benefits of the NingXia Wolfberry have been recognized for centuries. Although there are actually 17 different species of Wolfberries, the NingXia Wolfberry is the most nutritionally dense, and the most researched and tested Wolfberry on the market.
NingXia Red has documented health supporting properties and supports every system of the body which is why we have included it in every system throughout the book and each sample plan.

OmegaGize 3
OmegaGize 3 combines the benefits of three of the most essential supplements—omega-3 fatty acids, vitamin D-3, and CoQ10 (ubiquinone) which are enhanced with our proprietary essential oil blend to create an omega-3, DHA rich supplement that supports overall wellness. These ingredients work synergistically to support normal brain, heart, eye, and joint health.

Super C Chewables and Tablets
Provides 2,166% (that's not a typo) of the recommended daily intake of vitamin C and is fortified with natural electrolyte-balancing ingredients to promote optimum immune and circulatory function.

MultiGreens
Contains a chlorophyll based formula designed to boost vivacity by working with the glandular, nervous, and circulatory systems to relieve stress. This supplement promotes energy metabolism and glucose utilization. MultiGreens is made with spirulina, alfalfa sprouts, barley grass, bee pollen, eleuthero, Pacific kelp and Young Living Essential Oils.

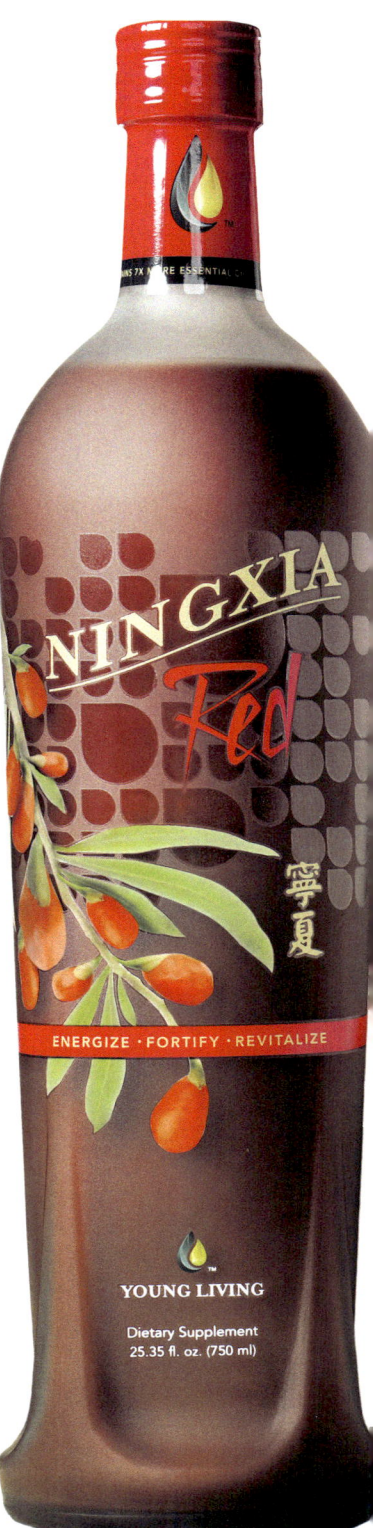

ROLLER BALL RECIPES

Seasonal Relief
- 3 drops Peppermint
- 3 drops Lemon
- 3 drops Lavender
- Carrier Oil

Relax
- 4 drops Orange
- 4 drops Stress Away
- Carrier Oil

Immune System Support
- 2 drops Lemon
- 2 drops Thieves
- 2 drops Tea Tree
- 2 drops Oregano
- 2 drops Frankincense
- Carrier Oil

Joint Support
- 4 drops Panaway
- 4 drops Copaiba
- Carrier Oil

Heatwave
- 5 drops Peppermint
- 2 drops Patchouli
- Carrier Oil

Peaceful Sleep
- 4 drops Stress Away
- 4 drops Lavender
- Carrier Oil

Tension-Filled Day
- 3 drops Frankincense
- 3 drops Peppermint
- 3 drops Lavender
- Carrier Oil

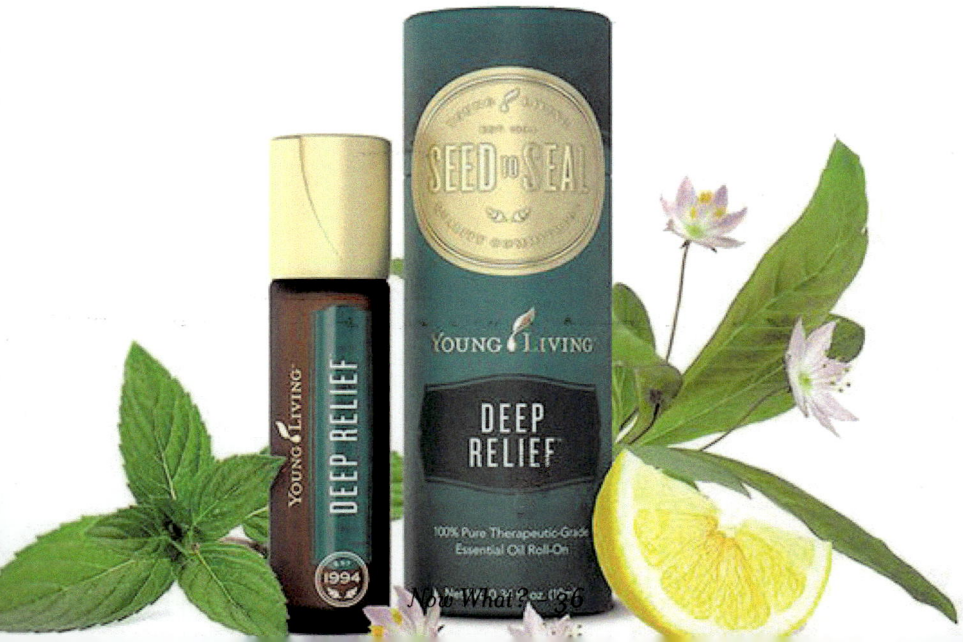

Silence
- 4 drops Orange
- 4 drops Cedarwood
- Carrier Oil

Motivation
- 3 drops Black Pepper
- 3 drops Lime
- 2 drops Orange
- 2 drops Frankincense
- Carrier Oil

Working Muscles
- 3 drops Peppermint
- 3 drops Clove
- 3 drops Wintergreen
- 2 drops Black Pepper
- Carrier Oil

Attentive
- 3 drops Vetiver
- 3 drops Cedarwood
- 3 drops Lavender
- Carrier Oil

Clear Brain
- 3 drops Rosemary
- 4 drops Lemon
- 2 drops Cypress
- Carrier Oil

Liquid Calm
- 3 drops Lavender
- 2 drops Valor
- 2 drops Stress Away
- 1 drop Patchouli
- 1 drop Vetiver
- Carrier Oil

Fountain of Youth
- 3 drops Frankincense
- 3 drops Lavender
- 3 drops Cypress
- Carrier Oil

Set the Mood
- 5 drops Ylang Ylang
- 2 drops Orange
- 2 drops Stress Away
- Carrier Oil

Carrier Oils:
- V-6 Vegetable Oil Complex by Young Living
- Fractionated Coconut Oil, Olive Oil, Grapeseed Oil, Jojoba Oil, Almond Oil

*All recipes are based on 10 ml size bottles.

DIFFUSER RECIPES

Seasonal Relief
- 2 drops Peppermint
- 2 drops Lemon
- 2 drops Lavender

Breath of Fresh Air
- 2 drops RC
- 2 drops Peppermint
- 2 drops Lemon

Stink-Be-Gone
- 6 drops Purification
- 2 drops Lemon

Strengthen and Purify
- 3 drops Thieves
- 3 drops Purification

Restful Sleep
- 4 drops Lavender
- 4 drops Cedarwood

Bedtime Peace
- 4 drops Stress Away
- 4 drops Lavender

Calm Air
- 2 drops Frankincense
- 2 drops Lavender
- 2 drops Stress Away

Reflections
- 3 drops Frankincense
- 2 drops Lemon

Mint Chocolate Chip
- 4 drops Stress Away
- 2 drops Peppermint

Bounce in My Step
- 4 drops Orange
- 2 drops Peppermint

Abundance
- 2 drops Abundance
- 4 drops Orange

Awake Brain
- 3 drops Peppermint
- 3 drops Rosemary

Shake it Off
- 3 drops Release
- 2 drops Peppermint

New Horizons
- 2 drops Abundance
- 2 drops Oola Finance
- 2 drops Oola Grow

Cheerful Focus
- 3 drops Cedarwood
- 3 drops Orange

My Happy Place
- 4 drops Orange
- 2 drops Abundance
- 2 drops Joy

Spring Freshness
- 2 drops Bergamot
- 2 drops Grapefruit
- 1 drop Ylang Ylang

Autumn Spice
- 2 drops Cinnamon Bark
- 2 drops Ginger
- 2 drops Orange

Pumpkin Spice
- 4 drops Cinnamon Bark
- 1 drop Clove
- 2 drops Nutmeg

Cozy by the Fire
- 3 drops Cinnamon Bark
- 2 drops Orange
- 1 drop Clove
- 1 drop Nutmeg

Winter Bliss
- 3 drops Christmas Spirit
- 2 drops Peppermint

Summer Fun
- 2 drops Bergamot
- 3 drops Oola Fun

Peaceful Sunset
- 2 drops Orange
- 1 drop Patchouli
- 1 drop Sandalwood
- 1 drop Ylang Ylang

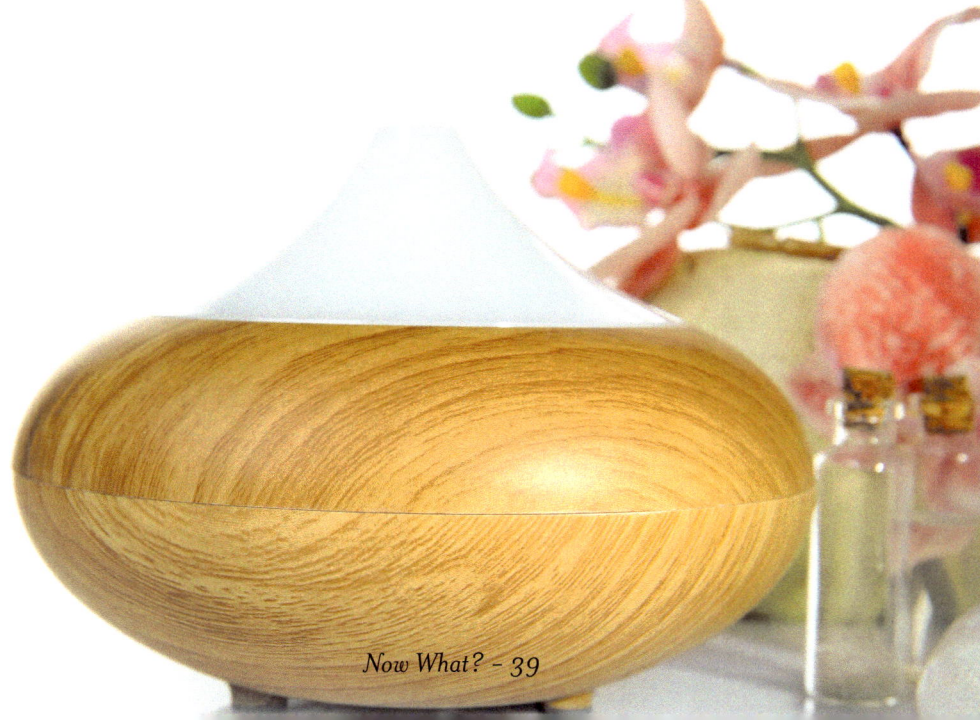

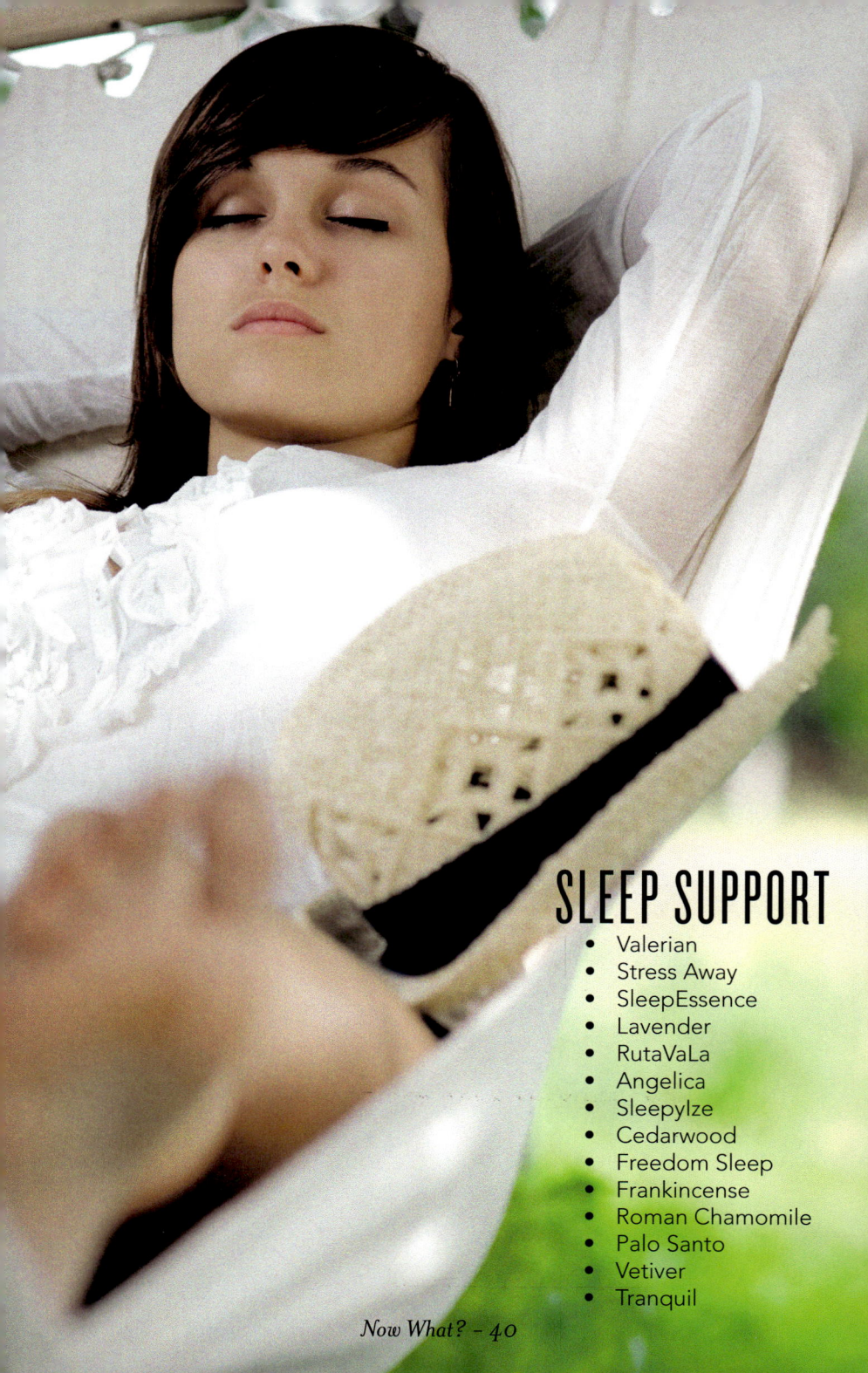

SLEEP SUPPORT

- Valerian
- Stress Away
- SleepEssence
- Lavender
- RutaVaLa
- Angelica
- SleepyIze
- Cedarwood
- Freedom Sleep
- Frankincense
- Roman Chamomile
- Palo Santo
- Vetiver
- Tranquil

KIDS SUPPORT

- Kidscents Bath Gel & Lotion
- Kidscents Tender Tush
- Kidscents Shampoo
- Kidscents Slique Toothpaste
- Kidscents MightyVites & MightyZymes
- Owie
- SniffleEase
- Frankincense
- TummyGize
- Gentle Baby
- Lavender
- The Reconnect Kit: GenYus, SleepyIze, Reconnect, InTouch

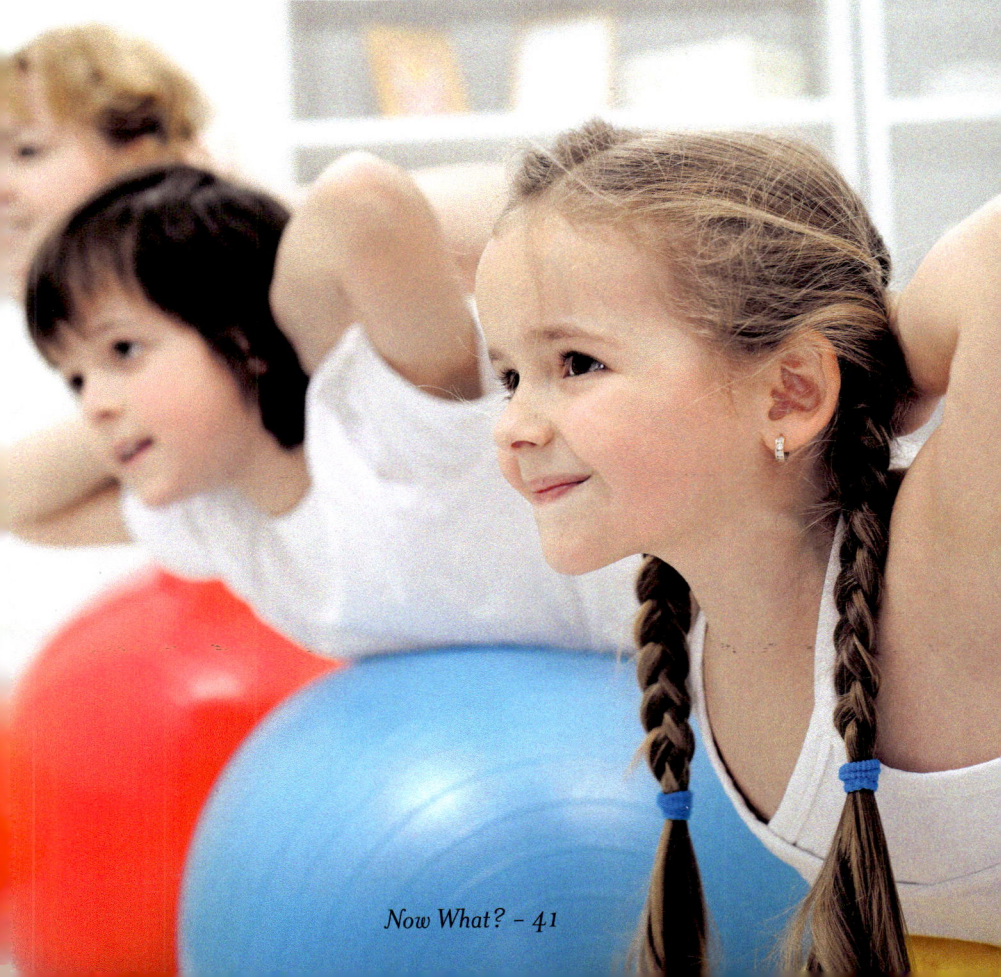

ENERGY/STAMINA

- Peppermint
- Palo Santo
- NingXia Red
- NingXia Nitro
- NingXia Zyng
- Citrus oils
- En-R-Gee
- Black Pepper
- PowerGize
- MultiGreens
- AminoWise
- SuperB

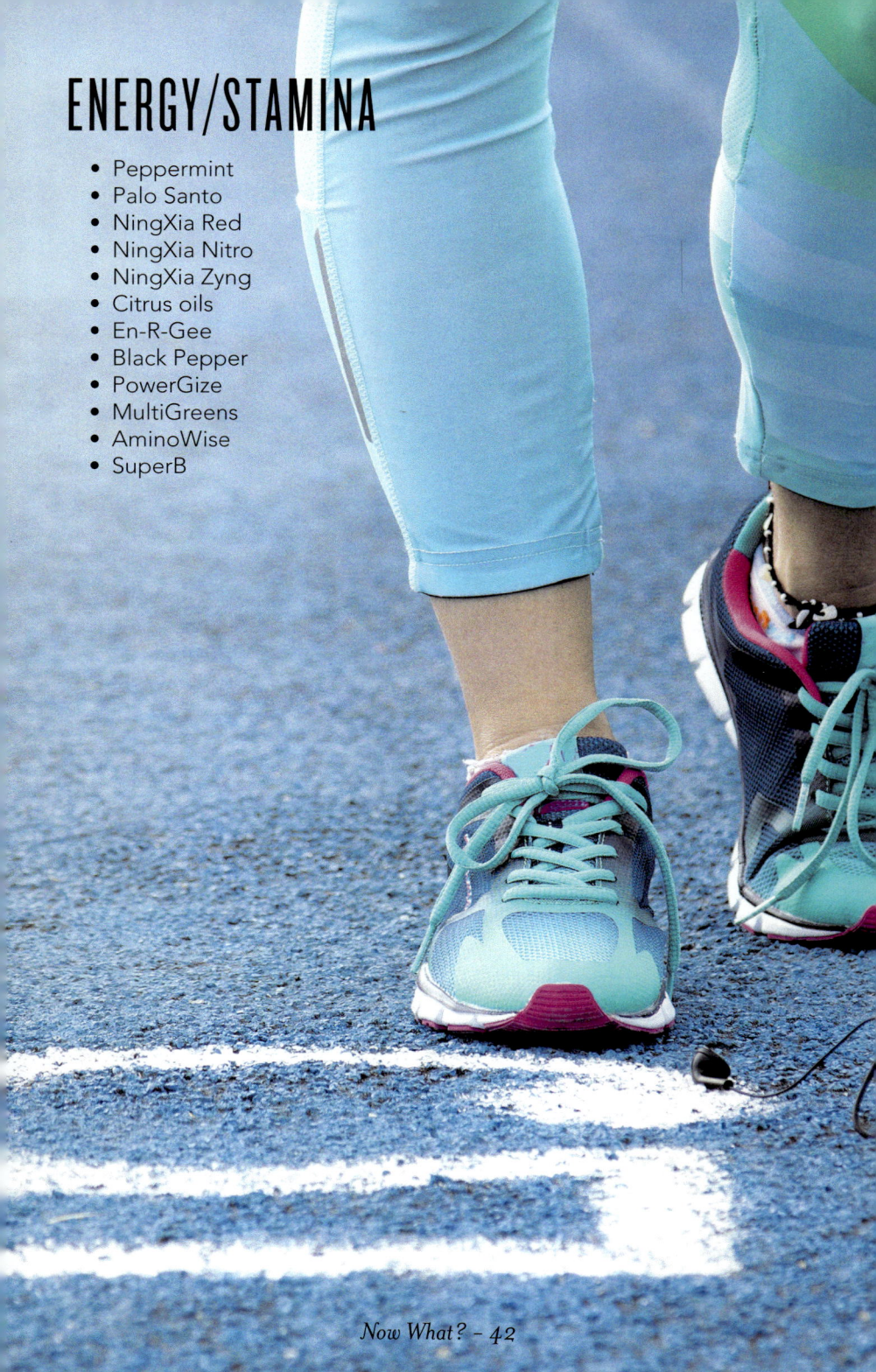

BRAIN HEALTH

- Frankincense
- Cedarwood
- Brain Power
- Clarity
- Sacred Sandalwood
- MindWise
- NingXia Red
- NingXia Nitro
- The Reconnect Kit: GenYus, SleepyIze, Reconnect, InTouch

*See also gastrointestinal and nervous systems

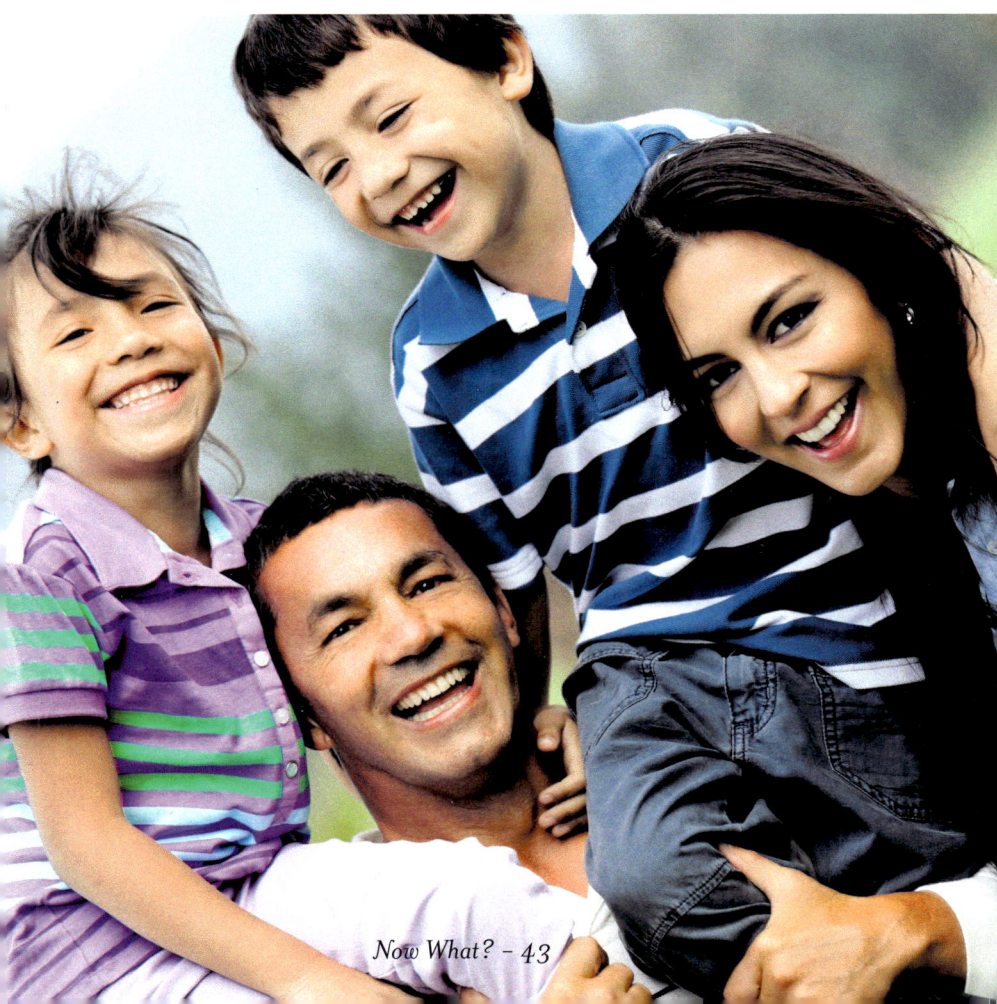

BABY SUPPORT

- Seedlings Diaper Rash Ointment
- Seedlings Baby Oil
- Seedlings Baby Wash & Shampoo
- Seedlings Baby Wipes
- Seedlings Linen Spray
- Lavender
- Gentle Baby
- Frankincense
- Myrrh
- Lemon
- Peace & Calming

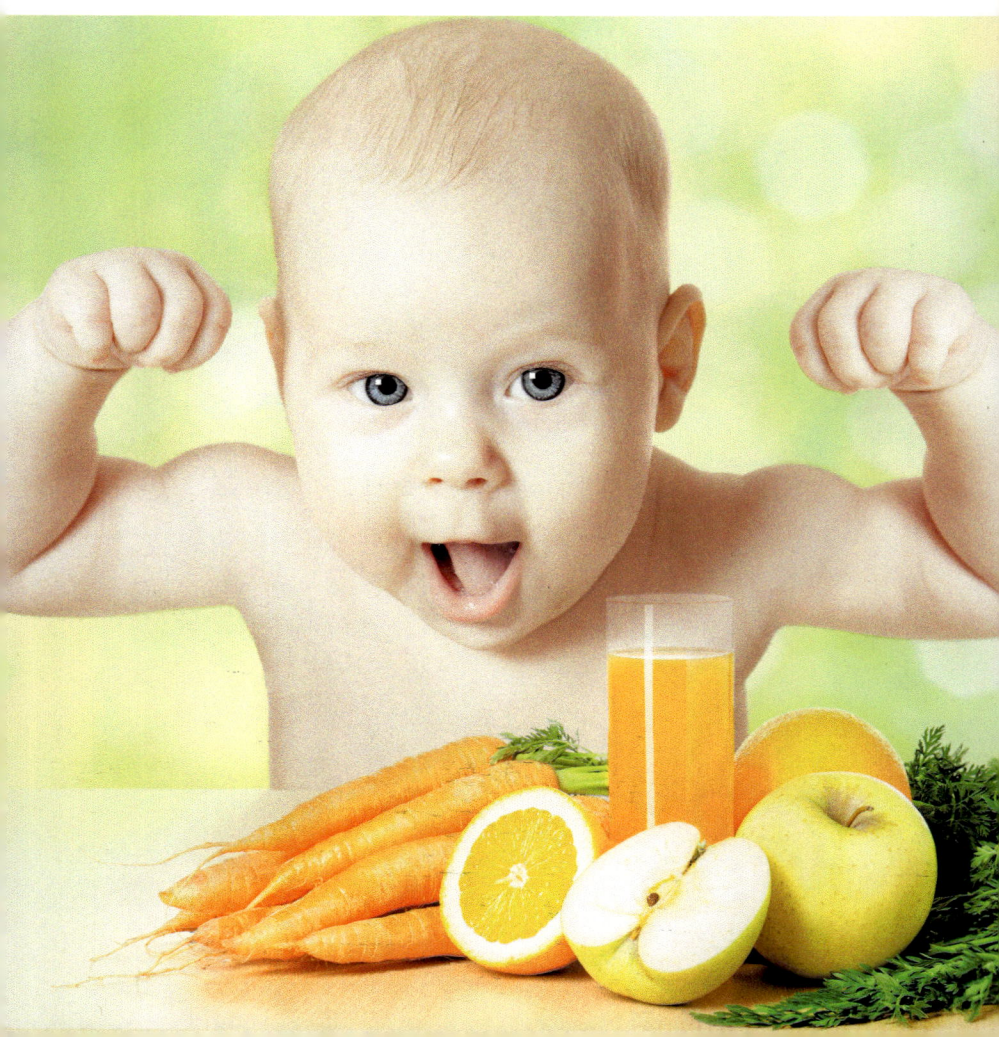

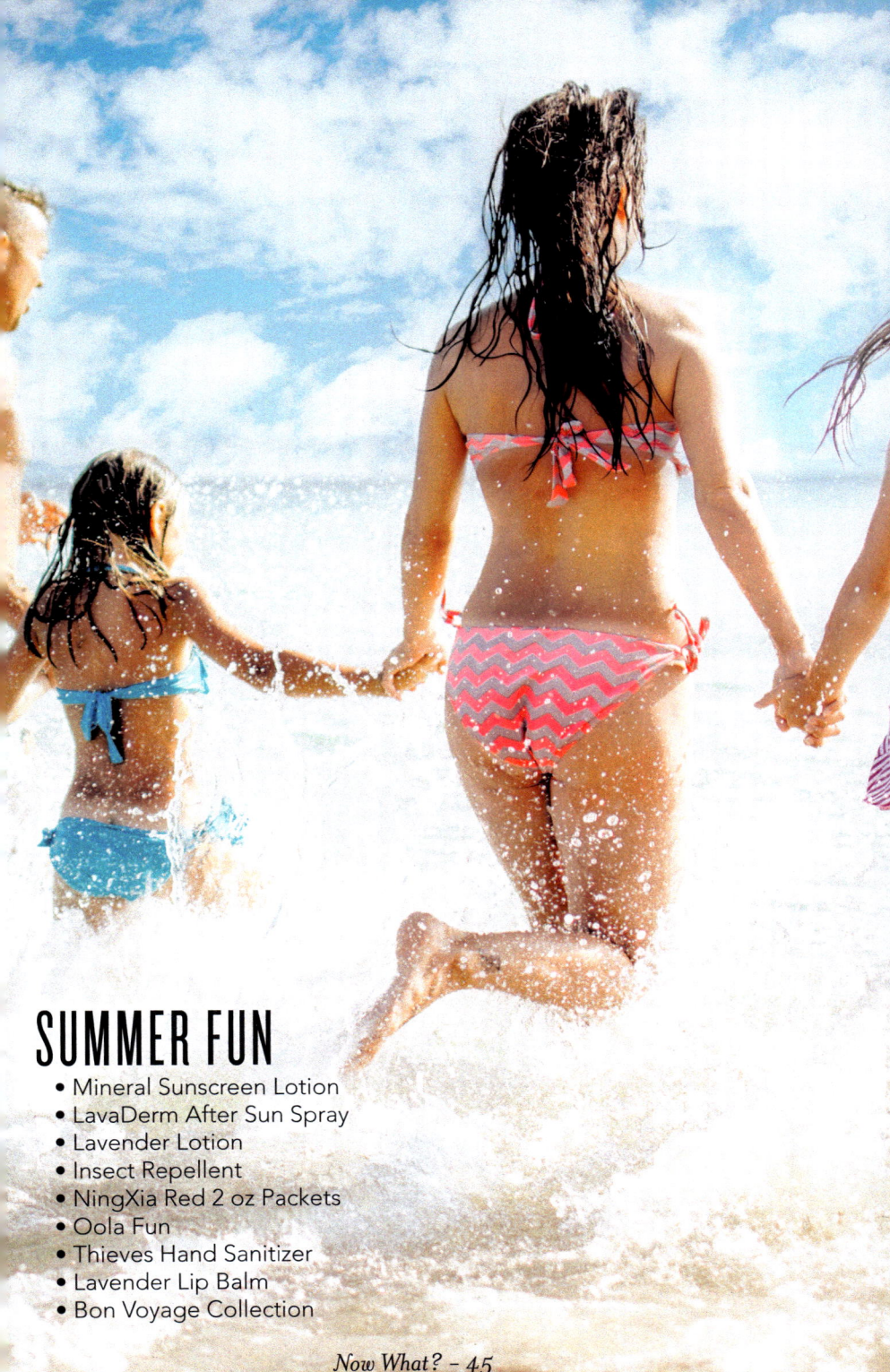

SUMMER FUN
- Mineral Sunscreen Lotion
- LavaDerm After Sun Spray
- Lavender Lotion
- Insect Repellent
- NingXia Red 2 oz Packets
- Oola Fun
- Thieves Hand Sanitizer
- Lavender Lip Balm
- Bon Voyage Collection

YOUNG LIVING MEMBERSHIP BENEFITS

Some of the unique benefits of a Young Living membership include:

- **Generous Compensation:** Young Living offers an industry leading compensation plan with generous commissions, bonuses, travel, and recognition.

- **Wholesale Pricing:** Save 24% off retail pricing. And save even more money with exclusive specials, our Essential Rewards program, and amazing promotions every month.

- **Essential Rewards**: As a member, you are eligible to enroll in the ER program and earn as much as 25% back in Reward Points toward free product. (See pages 5-6)

- **Exclusive Experiences:** Participate in unique events such as our annual International Grand Convention which is SO MUCH FUN. Also, check out Lavender Days at the Mona Utah Farm where you can experience our Seed to Seal® process firsthand. Ask your sponsor how to qualify for free global recognition retreats and leadership cruises.

- **Community:** Enjoy a close-knit community of support with your team and access your team's free ongoing training and Facebook resources. In addition to your sponsor, you have access to the entire Young Living family and we are all ready to assist and encourage you in your journey.

- **Education:** Young Living provides ongoing health education opportunities through conventions, seminars, and newsletters to keep you informed and assist you in your wellness progress.

- **Recognition:** As you expand your organization and advance toward the prestigious rank of Royal Crown Diamond, you will enjoy special recognition for your accomplishments and leadership!

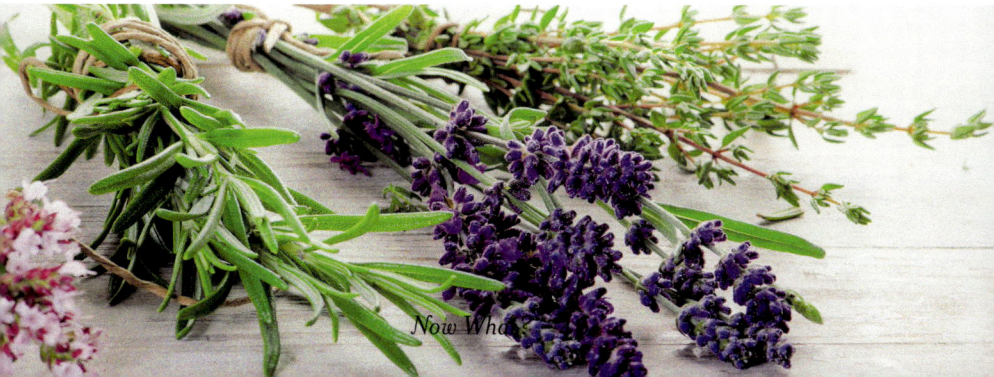

Now What

Young Living offers an amazing business opportunity and generous perks to membership…aside from improving the health of your family, friends, and YOU!

Do you want to truly own your time—and your life?
Wouldn't it be nice if going to work every day was fun and exciting?

Living paycheck to paycheck?
Wouldn't it be nice if you pay your bills with ease?

Young Living's generous compensation plan gives you the power to take control of your future, build your own business, and change your life forever.

Being a Young Living member goes beyond simply building a thriving business. We enjoy extensive networking opportunities, exclusive hands-on experiences, free ongoing training and support, as well as a strong sense of community.

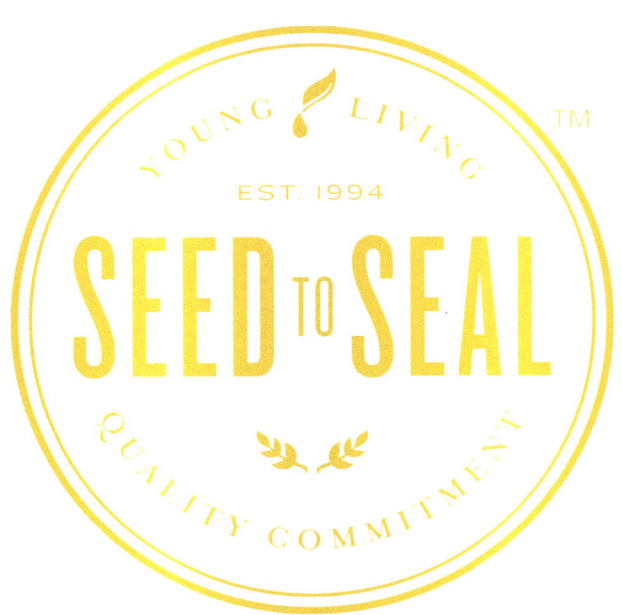

SHARE MORE...

Life Science Publishing and Products has everything you need to explore the history, the traditions, the research, the science, and the uses for all essential oils. Visit www.discoverlsp.com to learn how you can make the most of every essential oil single or blend. Whether you need books or tools for your home, glassware for your business, or brochures for helping you share, consider Life Science Publishing and Products your perfect partner.

© Life Science Publishing. All rights reserved. No part of this book may be reproduced or transmitted in any form or by any means, electronic or mechanical, including photocopying, recording, or by any information storage and retrieval system, without permission in writing from the publisher.

Content herein derives from the Essential Oil Desk Reference, also owned and published by Life Science Publishing.

Life Science Publishing is the publisher of this handbook. Life Science Publishing is not responsible for its content. The information contained herein is for educational purposes only. It is not provided to diagnose, prescribe, or treat any condition of the body. The information in this handbook should not be used as a substitute for medical counseling with a health professional. Neither the authors nor the publisher accepts responsibility for such use.